Complexity, Science and Society

Edited by

JAN BOGG

Academic Sub Dean, Medical Faculty,
University of Liverpool, UK
Co-Director, Centre for Complexity Research

and

ROBERT GEYER

Professor of Politics, Complexity and Policy
Department of Politics and International Relations,
Lancaster University, UK
Co-Director, Centre for Complexity Research

Radcliffe Publishing
Oxford • New York

Radcliffe Publishing Ltd
18 Marcham Road
Abingdon
Oxon OX14 1AA
United Kingdom

www.radcliffe-oxford.com
Electronic catalogue and worldwide online ordering facility.

British Library Cataloguing in Publication Data

A catalogue record for this book is available from the British Library.

ISBN-13: 978 1 84619 203 6

Typeset by 4word Ltd, Bristol
Printed and bound by TJ International Ltd, Padstow, Cornwall

Contents

List of contributors

Peter Allen is a professor at the Complex Systems Management Centre, School of Management, Cranfield University.

Pierpaolo Andriani is Senior Lecturer in Management of Innovation at Durham Business School, Durham University. His current research and publications focus on the impact on organisations of some theoretical aspects of complexity theory (such as power laws and fractals), the emergent properties of organisational networks (including industrial clusters) and distributed innovation. He is Visiting Scholar at several Universities including the Anderson School, University of California Los Angeles, University of Salento (Italy) and Udine (Italy).

Abbie Badcock is a graduate (in International Politics and Policy, from the School of Politics and Communications), University of Liverpool. Additionally, she worked part-time for the Centre for Complexity Research co-ordinating the 2005 conference. Her academic interests in political applications of complexity resulted in a comparative dissertation of political theory, globalisation and international terrorism.

Gert Biesta is Professor of Education at the Institute of Education, University of Stirling, Scotland, and Visiting Professor for Education and Democratic Citizenship at Örebro University, Sweden, and Mälardalen University, Sweden. Taking inspiration from pragmatism (Dewey, Mead) and post-structuralism (Derrida, Levinas), he conducts theoretical and empirical research on the many relationships between education and democracy.

Jan Bogg is Co-Director of the Centre for Complexity Research and is Director of the ESF-funded Breaking Barriers in the Workforce Project; she is also Academic Sub Dean of the Medical Faculty at the University of Liverpool, and Course Director for Behavioural Sciences for Allied Health Professionals. Jan is dual-qualified as an organisational and health psychologist; her organisational research specialises in NHS workforce issues. She holds a consultant psychologist honorary contract with a local NHS Trust, attached to the clinical practice and research unit. She is also editor of the British Psychological Society, Psychological Testing Centre, and in 2005 was elected to the International Test Council, which set standards and guidelines in psychometric testing.

Cary A. Brown, Lecturer, School of Health Sciences, University of Liverpool. Cary has had a range of clinical and academic experiences in Canada, the Middle East and the United Kingdom that informs her work in chronic pain.

Ceri Brown, Consultant in Anaesthesia and Intensive Care, North Manchester General Hospital. A practising clinician, interested in complexity and its application to health care for the past 10 years.

David Byrne is a Professor at the School of Applied Social Sciences, Durham University. His extensive research includes methodology, social exclusion and urban change.

Paul Cilliers is Professor of Philosophy at the University of Stellenbosch in South Africa. He also has a degree in Electronic Engineering but teaches mainly Cultural Philosophy and Deconstruction. His research is focused on the philosophical and ethical implications of complexity theory. He is the author of *Complexity and Postmodernism* (Routledge, 1998).

Anthony Grayham Deakin, Senior Research Associate, University of Liverpool. Member of the Centre for Intelligent Monitoring Systems, researching and developing chromatic technology to assist in the management of complex systems, particularly in medical, biological and electrical engineering domains.

Kingsley Dennis, Department of Sociology, Lancaster University. His current research examines complexity models for physical-digital social movements. Research interests also include complex mobilities, information communication technologies and digital cartographies. Upcoming research involves social uses of virtual worlds, geospace and networks of web applications.

Jean-Pierre Georgé, University Paul Sabatier, IRIT, France. Jean-Pierre is interested in co-operative self-organising mechanisms in multi-agent systems.

Carlos Gershenson is at the Centrum Leo Apostel, Vrije Universiteit Brussel. He is interested in self-organising systems, artificial life, evolution, complexity, cognition and artificial societies, and specialises in philosophy.

Robert Geyer is Professor of Politics, Complexity and Policy in the Department of Politics and International Relations at Lancaster University, and is Co-Director of the Centre for Complexity Research. His works include *Exploring European Social Policy* (2000) (co-authored with Andrew Mackintosh), *Integrating UK and European Social Policy: The complexity of Europeanisation* (2005), and (co-authored with Helen Cooper) *Riding the Diabetes Rollercoaster: A new approach for health professionals, patients and carers* (2007).

Marie-Pierre Gleizes, University Paul Sabatier, IRIT, France. Marie-Pierre is interested in methodologies and tools for the design of adaptive multi-agent systems.

Pierre Glize, University Paul Sabatier, IRIT, France. He is interested in the study of emergence in complex artificial systems.

Gustavo Gomes de Freitas, Complex – University of São Paulo, Brazil. Themes of interest: economies as evolutionary and decentralised many-body systems analysed by statistical and computational approaches.

Tamsin Haggis is Lecturer in Lifelong Learning at the Institute of Education, University of Stirling, Scotland. Her research focuses on the different ways that learning is defined, researched and theorised, particularly within the field of Higher Education. More generally, she is exploring the possibilities of complexity and dynamic systems theories in relation to theory, epistemology and method in educational research.

Paul Haynes, Skoll Centre, Said Business School, Oxford University. Uses complexity to explore the relationship between innovation and social change. Research interests include entrepreneurship, networks and technology.

Francis Heylighen is research professor at the Vrije Universiteit Brussel, where he leads the Evolution, Complexity and Cognition research group, affiliated with the interdisciplinary Center Leo Apostel. He is editor of the Principia Cybernetica website (pcp.vub.ac.be), which develops an evolutionary-cybernetic philosophy. His interests are focused mainly on the emergence of intelligent organisation in complex systems.

Tim Holt is a Clinical Lecturer at the Health Sciences Research Institute, Warwick Medical School. Tim is an academic general practitioner with a research interest in complexity theory applied to information technology and diabetes care.

Tammy Iftody is a Doctoral candidate at the University of British Columbia. Tammy's research interests include studies in consciousness and popular culture. Currently, she is looking into the ways in which popular forms of narrative (i.e. memoir, docu-drama, reality television) reflect new understandings about the relationship between human consciousness, identity and imagination.

Andrew Innes, General Practitioner, Church View Surgery, Hedon, East Yorkshire. Dr Innes is a general practitioner and research fellow at the University of Hull. His research interest is in the consultation as a complex system.

Pejman Iravani, Research Fellow, Robotics and Intelligent Systems Design, the Open University, UK. Pejman is interested in intelligent adaptive systems and the application of hypernetworks in team robotics and multiagent systems.

Bob Jessop, Director of the Institute for Advanced Studies, Lancaster University. He is best known for his contributions to state theory, political economy, the regulation approach and the philosophy of social sciences.

Jeffrey Johnson, Research Professor of Complexity Science and Design, Open University, UK. Research is on the development of the mathematical theory of hypernetworks for multilevel system dynamics in the science of complex physical, human and socio-technical systems. Jeffrey sees multi-agent modelling as an important development in the science of complex systems.

Gordon Rees Jones, Emeritus Professor, Senior Research Fellow, University of Liverpool. Founder and past director of the Centre for Intelligent Monitoring Systems for advancing research into the use of chromatic methodologies to extract information about complex situations/systems ranging from electric arc plasma to medical conditions.

Rod Lambert, Lecturer, School of Allied Health Professions, Institute of Health, University of East Anglia, Norwich. University lecturer and Director of Post-Graduate Taught Programmes. Rod has an interest in examining how complexity science can inform current concepts and clinical applications in mental health.

Kai Lehmann is a PhD candidate at the University of Liverpool. He also works as a Visiting Lecturer at the University of Greenwich. He teaches International and European Union Politics. His research interests include international relations theory and foreign policy decision-making processes.

Rebecca Luce-Kapler is Professor of Language and Literacy in the Faculty of Education, Queen's University, Kingston, Ontario, Canada. Her research and work focus on writing processes and technologies. In 2004, Lawrence Erlbaum published her book *Writing With, Through and Beyond the Text: An ecology of language*.

Paul Marrow, Pervasive ICT Research Centre, BT Group plc, UK. Paul is interested in nature-inspired computing and the complexity of natural systems, multi-agent systems, the control of decentralised systems, and complex systems in healthcare.

Carmel M. Martin, Associate Professor of Family Medicine, Northern Ontario School of Medicine, Ontario, Canada. Carmel, general practitioner and researcher, has specialised in the development and evaluation of primary care reforms in the UK, Australia and Canada.

Peter McBurney, Department of Computer Science, University of Liverpool. Peter's interests lie in agent-based modelling and simulation, agent communication languages, interaction protocols, and automated mechanism design.

Elizabeth McMillan, Senior Research Fellow, the Open University, co-founder and a Director of the Complexity Society UK. Research interests: complexity – strategy, change, innovation, organisational dynamics and design. Book: *Complexity, Organizations and Change*.

Yasmin Merali, Director, Information Systems Research Unit, Warwick Business School, University of Warwick, Coventry. Yasmin has extensive consultancy experience, advising on management of business transformation programmes in the network economy. She has developed the 'information lens' to explore transformational dynamics, and her current research is on the use of complexity theory to study organisation in the information space.

Deborah Osberg is a postdoctoral fellow in the School of Education and Lifelong Learning at the University of Exeter, England. With an MSc in Zoology (evolutionary ecology) and a PhD in Educational Theory, she uses complexity as an organising framework to explore the implications of dynamically relational theoretical forms for educational theory and practice.

Jeremy Andrew Leslie Rabone, Graduate Research Student, Birkbeck College, London. Computational Chemist (MChem, Oxon) with an interest in programming cellular automata and chemical simulation.

Jonathan Kenneth Rabone, Director Four Delta Consulting Ltd, Edinburgh. A software engineer (M. Eng, MA, Cantab) with an interest in programming cellular automata.

Kenneth Leslie Rabone, Senior Fellow, Department of Physics, University of Liverpool, formerly Unilever Research. Experienced in the formulation of novel, hygienic cleaners through design-driven use of high-throughput experimentation

Samir Rihani, Research Fellow, University of Liverpool, Department of Politics and Communication Studies. Works on complex systems following work in transportation planning. Experienced NHS non-executive director. Author of *Complex Systems Theory and Development Practice*. Professional and academic work focuses mainly on human and economic development.

Joseph William Spencer, University of Liverpool. Current director of the Centre for Intelligent Monitoring Systems, with research interests on using the chromatic method for information extraction and the detection of emergent patterns.

Joachim P. Sturmberg, Professor of General Practice; Department of General Practice, Monash University, Australia, and Department of General Practice, Newcastle University, Newcastle, Australia. His research interests relate to the exploration of health as an individual construct, and how this value drives the planning provision and outcomes of the health service.

Dennis Sumara, Professor and Head of Curriculum Studies at the University of British Columbia, Canada. He conducts research into imaginative engagement in contexts of learning and teaching, with specific attention to how literary forms mediate and condition the ongoing emergence of human consciousness. His latest book, *Why Reading Literature in School Still Matters: Imagination, interpretation, insight*, won the 2003 National Reading Conference Ed Fry Book Award.

Gilberto Tadeu Lima, Department of Economics, University of São Paulo, Brazil. He is interested in agent-based modelling and simulation of evolutionary, complex macrodynamic behaviour.

Martin Watson, Senior Lecturer, School of Allied Health Professions, Institute of Health, University of East Anglia, Norwich, UK. University lecturer and course director with clinical, teaching and research interests in physical therapy treatment of movement disorders caused by acquired brain injuries.

Adam Wellstead, Natural Resources Canada-Canadian Forest Service, Northern Forestry Centre, Edmonton, Alberta, Canada. MA (political science), MSc (forestry), PhD (renewable resources with a specialisation in public policy). Research interests include quantitative methods in policy research, organisational research, and understanding policy capacity.

Mateo Willis is an artist and independent filmmaker with a particular interest in complexity. Samples of his work can be seen at www.mateowillis.com.

CHAPTER 1

Introduction

Robert Geyer and Jan Bogg

In his most famous work, *The Communist Manifesto*, Karl Marx proclaimed that 'a spectre is haunting Europe – the spectre of Communism'. We want to claim that a new spectre is haunting Europe and beyond: the spectre of complexity. Our claim may not be wrapped in so flowery and revolutionary prose, but the long-term impact of complexity thinking on the fundamental understanding of our natural and social worlds may be even more radical and revolutionary. For both of us, complexity thinking has drastically reshaped our perceptions of our own fields, the nature of higher education, interactions between academic disciplines, the constraints and potential of public policy and the role of social systems in human development. In essence, we have undergone a so-called 'paradigm shift' in our own thinking. Or, as the Nobel Prize winning Ilya Prigogine eloquently argued:

> *'We believe that we are actually at the beginning of a new scientific era. We are observing the birth of a science that is no longer limited to idealized and simplified situations but reflects the complexity of the real world, a science that views us and our creativity as part of a fundamental trend present at all levels of nature'* [1].

What is complexity and how has it developed as an academic discipline?

We see complexity as a broad term for describing and understanding a wide range of chaotic, dissipative, adaptive, nonlinear and complex systems and phenomena. Emerging out of the physical sciences in the early to mid-20th century and increasingly spilling over into the social sciences at the end of that century, complexity is a new and exciting interdisciplinary approach to science and society that challenges traditional academic divisions, frameworks and paradigms.

Until recent decades, many of the discoveries in the natural sciences were formulated within a linear paradigm that emerged during the Enlightenment. Descartes and Newton were the principal architects of the new paradigm: the former advocated intellectual rationalism, whereas the latter presented a whole raft of fundamental physical laws. Given this belief in human rationality and fundamental physical order, there seemed to be no limit to the ability of human beings to comprehend and hence control the natural world. The phenomenal success of the Industrial Revolution was built on this paradigm.

However, during the 20th century the natural sciences began to experience a Kuhnian 'paradigm shift' that propelled them beyond the confines of the Newtonian linear paradigm. The extraordinary mathematical work of Henri Poincaré, insights into the butterfly effect of the American meteorologist Edward Lorenz, Nobel Prize-winning work of physicist Murray Gell-Man, biological studies of Stuart Kauffman at the Santa Fe Institute and work of many others probed and then expanded the limits set by Newton and Descartes.

Not surprisingly, the earlier success of the linear paradigm in the natural sciences had a profound effect on the social sciences. Surrounded by the technological marvels of the Industrial Revolution, it did not take much of an intellectual leap to apply the lessons of the physical sciences to the social realm. Adam Smith and David Ricardo claimed to have captured the laws of economic interaction. Karl Marx wedded his vision of class struggle to an analysis of the capitalist mode of production to create the 'immutable' and deterministic laws of capitalist development. Economics, politics, sociology all became 'sciences', desperate to duplicate the success of the natural sciences. Moreover, this desire was institutionalised through the development of modern universities that created and reinforced the disciplinarisation and professionalisation of the social sciences [2].

Using the Newtonian frame of reference, modern social scientists assumed that physical and social phenomena were primarily linear and therefore predictable, orderly and would reach stable endpoints. The notable international success of Francis Fukuyama's book, *The End of History and the Last Man* (1993), which claimed that history had reached its endpoint, demonstrates the enduring attraction of the linear framework. However, in the past two decades complexity has begun to permeate the social sciences as well. Like the transformation in the natural sciences, the complexity paradigm does not disprove linear social science, but argues that there is a range of social phenomena beyond the boundaries of that framework. For the social sciences, complexity acts like a bridging strategy between order and disorder and significantly refocuses the basis for understanding social life and state action. Instead of searching for and trying to impose some type of final order (be that a new 'Third Way' or a 'new and improved' health system), researchers and policy practitioners are starting to look for ways of promoting complex interactions and systems for enhancing rather than eliminating complexity.

How did the 2005 Complexity, Science and Society Conference emerge and what did we learn?

Excited by the growing potential of complexity for public policy and the social sciences and as a tactic for breaking down the barriers between the social and natural sciences, Robert Geyer and Samir Rihani founded the Complexity Network (CN) in January 2002. It was designed as an informal network to promote complexity theories and applications in the University of Liverpool and Merseyside region, and increase symbiotic linkages between regional, national and international complexity organisations and activities. Its first meeting attracted academics from 20 different departments, the most interdisciplinary event that many of the participants had ever attended. Subsequently, the CN organised a website and held a conference, 'Introducing Complexity', in April 2002, which attracted participants from 35 different academic departments as well as several other business and governmental representatives.

Building on the success of the CN, the Centre for Complexity Research (CCR) was created in April 2003, directed by Robert Geyer. Jan Bogg joined as Co-Director in October 2004 and the CCR instigated several complexity-related events and began supporting various complexity research projects and initiatives. Meanwhile, the CN continued to grow to over 750 members from every major academic discipline in 45 different countries.

In 2003, we began planning for the 2005 Complexity, Science and Society (CSS) conference. We knew what we wanted, a major international event that would show the unique interdisciplinary power of complexity, but we did not really know what it would look like. Our first step was to organise subject coordinators who could provide the necessary linkages to the different disciplines. During 2003 and 2004, subject areas began to solidify, a conference website was put together and all of the detailed work of planning the conference venue and accommodation began. The conference was very successful, attracting over 400 participants in 18 subject areas from 30 different countries. Full conference details are available at www.liv.ac.uk/ccr.

Conference evaluations were very positive and we learned several key lessons about organising interdisciplinary complexity conferences, including:

- Subject coordinators are the real strength of a successful conference. Like any complex system they must be given general parameters and then allowed to develop their own strategies. Some will fail and some will succeed. Accepting that inevitable unevenness is part of the process.
- Different disciplines have different academic 'currencies'. We were constantly surprised by the different social norms and tactics of different disciplines. From the need to publish conference papers, to organisational structures, to approaches to conference pricing (some wanted high conference registration fees to attract 'respect' for the conference), each discipline had distinctive aspects that needed to be integrated or compromised.
- Linking activities are essential. To encourage interdisciplinary interaction we kept the daily sessions to a minimum and allowed for plenty of 'coffee time', hosted daily plenary sessions and organised coordinated social events. However, we could have done more with 'break out' sessions, open workshops or even assigning people to take part in the activities of unrelated disciplines.
- Get the basics right, but don't forget about the little things. We were very happy with the basic structure of the conference, but as some of the evaluations pointed out, what people often remember is the little things. Is the coffee good? Were the biscuits nice? It was amazing how much these things mattered. In essence, the butterfly effect still counts even at conferences.

And the results

Of the 18 subject areas, we selected nine to include in the book as a 'taster' of what the conference was like. We asked the subject coordinators to choose the papers that were interesting, groundbreaking and accessible to as wide an audience as possible.

Obviously, these aspects are not all mutually compatible, but the following sections are a very good representation of the core developments of complexity thinking in several major fields. We realise that not all chapters will be of equal interest to every reader. However, our intention was to provide an accessible interdisciplinary introduction to the wonderful intellectual breadth that complexity can offer. Moreover, we sincerely hope that some of the excitement that we felt at the conference has carried over into the book. In some small way, we hope that this book will help to bring about what Stephen Hawking said in early 2000:

> *'I believe the next century will be the century of complexity'* [3].

References

1. Prigogine I. *The End of Certainty: Time, chaos and the new laws of nature.* New York: Free Press. 1997.
2. Gulbenkian Commission. *Open the Social Sciences: Report of the Gulbenkian Commission on the Restructuring of the Social Sciences.* Stanford: Stanford University Press. 1996.
3. See www.comdig.org.

CHAPTER 2

Art and complexity: complexity from the outside

Mateo Willis

> '*Mixture is greatness*'—SPANISH SAYING

It is perhaps our ability as human beings to differentiate that provides us with our unique mental capabilities, setting us apart from the other animals. Whether as a scientist sifting through data or a child learning to spell, we use the faculty to sort and categorise. As a strategy in a complicated world, this ability to short-hand our environment is incredibly useful. By reducing the detail level, we minimise the amount of energy-intensive thinking needed to make the right decisions. But an accurate picture of reality is probably more complicated than we can even imagine.

Let's face it, the world is a scary place, filled with much that is unknown and sometimes unknowable. For most of human existence we have been trying to stamp out this uncertainty through the generation of rules, laws, methods, religion

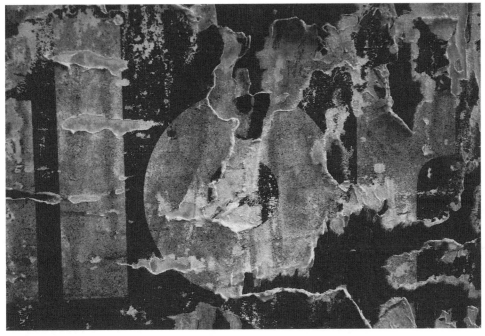

Figure 2.1. Poster.

and scientific principles. But none of these procedures has completely tamed the uncertain and reductionism often falls short of an adequate explanation. The theories of complexity make up a loose collection of tools that approach this problem from a new angle, useful not just from a scientific perspective but also from the arts, enabling the creation of alternative and hopefully improved models of reality.

To find an example of a complex process one need look no further than the definition of the theory of complexity. When I first stumbled across the topic I spent months trying to pin down what the term meant. As an artist I was starting with a blank slate as my discipline did not have a canon of complexity research behind it, nor was there much of a peer group actively using these theories as part of their work. Every definition I searched for had a slightly different label. The biologists and physicists, sociologists and urban planners I spoke to interpreted it in a manner relative to their own domain. There was much overlap between disciplines but it was interesting to observe the way in which each individual bent it to their own needs, using it to illuminate their own concerns, be those economics, health care, philosophy, chemistry, design or engineering. It was an emergent definition shaped by multiple interactions.

This fluidity of definition can be both a strength and weakness. On the one hand it can be used in a variety of situations to expand explanation. Rather like a living, breathing language, it is malleable to the needs of the moment and this flexibility could lend it longevity. But complexity as a term only has strength if it does not become too blurred, attached to anything that is slightly complicated and thereby stripping it of its veracity. If that does become the case we will soon see complexity going the way of Esperanto or theosophy, movements that attracted initial followings but failed to live up to their promises.

How does this patchwork of a theory, 'complexity', relate to art? Art is a component of the way that we see the world. As part of our primitive intelligence's inability to fully comprehend reality, we translate what we see into caricatures and we enjoy sharing this product of our natural curiosity. This personal and biased outlook is the combination of multiple experiences, informed through a continual feedback loop with our environment. Art taps into this cycle and manifests those essences that drip through, solidifying emotions and experiences. Art, something that often exists outside of quantifiable logic, is not only created through a complex, adaptive process. Like circles within circles within circles, the theories of complexity can be seen in action within the entire art world.

The creation, business, appreciation and academic study of art exists in a state far from equilibrium. The system demands variations from artists who inevitably search for their own voice, innovation is applauded, prices fluctuate and trends change. It is an open system with energy that flows in and dissipates, fuelling the creation of work. The art world lurches from movement to movement, as fashions and styles become popular, then end up either forgotten or consigned to art history. These change unpredictably due to a large number of small units acting as individuals within the phase space of behaviour. The art world is constantly evolving, creating its own structures then devouring them and rolling on.

I like to imagine it is similar to Per Bak's [1] famous hypothetical sand pile. Imagine the scenario: tension builds up as artists, galleries and critics start to accept and attach labels to a certain style of art. This creates a feedback loop which

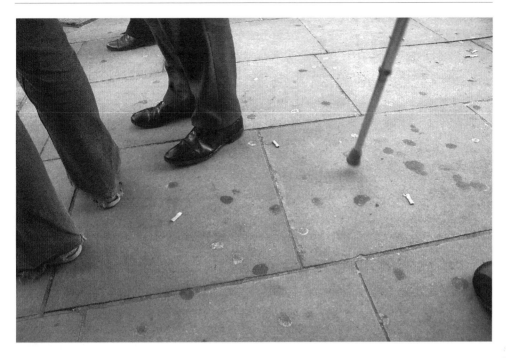

Figure 2.2. Pavement.

encourages those that fit within the mould to produce more work until a point of critical mass is reached and it becomes a publicly recognised style. This is the point of collapse. Once a movement has a label, a particular 'ism', anything new created after it is a move away from the original starting point until one day it is put into a category of its own. This is the rebuilding of the sand pile. Impressionism morphed into Post-Impressionism, which in turn blasted the doors open onto Cubism, Expressionism and Abstraction.

Calling the arrival of an art movement a collapse may seem strange, but the system under which art is created and then consumed encourages a constant stream of new work, ideas and concepts. Scientifically it would be termed an open system: energy flows into it in the form of money, creativity and the artist's desire to create art. This is kept in a permanent state of non-equilibrium by the fact that art is sold, fashions change and people demand the shock of something new. Art is self-evolutionary; artists quite often develop their styles and explore new methods while building upon what has been done before. Picasso once famously remarked that there was no point in making art like cakes, each piece an exact imitation of its predecessor.

The art world also displays other characteristics of a dynamic system. It is the epitome of a small-world network, with dense interconnections between artists, dealers, teachers and critics, facilitating not only the transfer of art but also the dissemination of ideas and concepts that slowly roll the art world along. A quote from the popular science writer Mark Buchanan provides an apt overview of the process:

'Self-organised criticality seems to show up only in things that are driven very slowly away from equilibrium, and in which the actions of any individual piece are dominated by its interactions with other elements' [2].

Although the parallels I make here are unscientific to the extreme, I believe that there is some value in examining the art world in this way.

Steven Strogatz, in his book *Sync* [3], claims that people have an inbuilt sense of periodicity and therefore respond well to physical and temporal patterns. I think this extends deeply into our behaviour, that we are susceptible to patterns that we are not even consciously aware of. A very physical example was the opening of the Millennium Bridge in London in 2000. The crowd walking on it caused the bridge to sway from side to side. Many pedestrians fell spontaneously into step with the bridge's vibrations, which had the effect of inadvertently amplifying the swing until it became physically perceptible and the bridge was closed for redesign three days later. Other examples are circadian rhythms or lunar cycles. These are all subtle (and not so subtle) influences, pushing us in one direction or another.

Artists' work often explores these subtle currents that weave their way between the pillars of logic and reason, without recourse to excessive explanation, rather like glimpsing sight of a distant star out of the corner of one's eye. I use complexity as a tool in my work, as part of the creation process as well as the filter through which I 'internalise' my experiences. An artistic viewpoint does not predicate 'truth': that is the job of science. Instead it is about experience, filtering out the extraneous and leaving behind the underlying essence of a particular focus. My work concentrates on

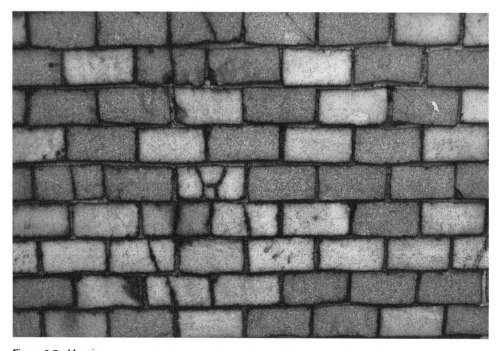

Figure 2.3. Mosaic.

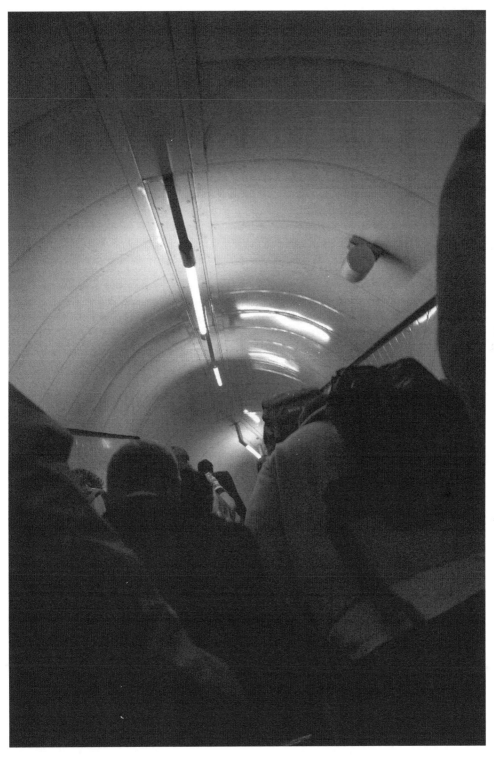

Figure 2.4. Tunnel.

massed humanity, particularly people in cities. This dense clustering yields forms of behaviour that is often only seen when in the close proximity of others.

Working with film and photography, I explore certain facets of busy streets, crowds, riots; situations of turmoil [4, 5]. Although my work seeks to reveal fragments, rather like the collected shards of a broken window, it does not attempt to put them back together and provide the full picture nor a descriptive illustration.

Complexity is useful as a tool because it allows an artist to dig deeper into the experience of the moment. Take some of the basic elements talked about in complexity theory and draw a direct analogy with a cluster of people: multiple connections, bifurcation points, adaptive emergence, constant change through the introduction of energy. As I am observing a crowd, which can range from a political demonstration to the aftermath of the London tube attacks, the metaphors allow me to absorb the dynamic as a whole. By using groups of people as a palette, I am then able to draw on opposing or complementary 'colours' to create unusual and hopefully insightful contrasts.

Through using complexity, I have found myself exploring what I term the negative space around people rather than the individuals themselves. To paraphrase and twist the words of the historian Edward Hallett Carr: art is not about the individual but rather the relationships between the individuals in society and the social forces that produce their actions [6]. It is this relationship between people, rather than the individuals themselves, that fascinates me. In the crowded, organic cities like Delhi and London, which bear their deeply layered past like a grubby overcoat, the incredible scale of interactions create multiple layers of emergent patterns. Millions of people moderate and change each other's behaviour and environment.

As much as we study the world around us, endlessly analysing and creating models of complex and intricate systems, I wonder if we will ever truly come to understand ourselves. If we can, part of that answer will lie with science. But some of our understanding will also be through art. It is not enough to use our unique, human ability to accurately categorise this world. It also has to be experienced.

References

1. Kauffman S. *At Home in the Universe*. London: Viking. 1995.
2. Buchanan B. *Ubiquity*. London: Phoenix. 2000.
3. Strogatz S. *Sync*. New York: Penguin. 2003.
4. Willis, M. London. *ca.* 2004. available from http://mateowillis.com/menupages/art/2EYESopen/2eyesopen.htm.
5. Willis, M. London. *ca.* 2006. available from http://mateowillis.com/menupages/art/21705/217051.html.
6. Carr, EH. *What is History?* New York: Knopf. 1962.

CHAPTER 3

Diversity, interconnectivity and sustainability

Peter M. Allen and Pierpaolo Andriani

Introduction

Over recent years, studies in complex systems and their structural evolution have shown that diversity is a key aspect in explaining their functioning and their co-operative and competitive interactions. However, what has been only poorly understood has been the importance of the diversity corresponding to different levels of description of a system. The species diversity that is present in an ecosystem is actually its functional structure – with different species filling different roles in the food webs – but this is the result of the differential amplification and suppression of lower level, individual micro-diversity, generated by all kinds of genetic, developmental and environmental factors. The other important point is that an ecosystem does not really have a 'functional' structure because it does not have a 'function'. Selection is purely on the basis of individual survival and not ecosystem performance. This implies that 'diversity' is an important feature of complex, evolutionary systems. It is both the 'driver' of evolution and also the outcome [1]. This involves both the 'selective' effects of interactions between species and the simultaneous mechanisms underlying micro-diversity that *discover* new 'strategies' or 'niches'. In biological thinking the micro-diversity that occurs is generally considered to be 'random' and independent of the selection processes that follow, whereas in human innovation we like to think that there is rational intention, calculation and belief that may 'channel' diversity into some narrower range. But in reality, rational intention can only drive ideas that are well understood already, and so characterise the development and exploitation of existing ideas, but new ideas and radical innovations are generally emergent and unexpected, leading into new areas and concerns, changing the goals, aims and values of people and changing their view of reality.

The session that took place at the Liverpool conference had a wide variety of speakers who contributed to a discussion of the role and importance of diversity within complex systems. These covered a wide variety of domains from the biological to the problems of business and industry, including organic food, shop building and a wide range of contexts where these ideas are important. The presentations involved philosophy, discourse, biology and ecology, human systems, organic farming, economics, business systems and urban development. This breadth demonstrates the fundamental importance of the concept of diversity and its role in evolutionary processes. Rather than select just two or three of the papers, we decided to provide a mixture of brief summaries of different presentations and contributions.

Philosophy

Diversity, identity and complexity

The first contribution came from Paul Cilliers, whose interest was in diversity and how it affects issues of difference, identity and complexity. Over the past few decades the notions of difference and diversity has received a lot of attention, especially in the social sciences. The underlying philosophical characteristics of the notion have, however, not always received sufficient scrutiny. In structuralist and post-structuralist theories of language, difference is the source of meaning. Similarly, in complex systems, difference, and the related notion of asymmetry, is responsible for the structural characteristics of such systems. It is therefore important to understand the 'logic' of this notion. The paper explored this by looking at several problems. The play of difference cannot generate specific meaning if differences reverberate infinitely. Meaning, albeit meaning that is constantly shifting, only comes to be under bounded conditions. There has to be a certain 'economy of difference'. Furthermore, we cannot use the notion of difference without reference to the notion of identity. Identity, however, does not determine difference: it is a result thereof. Complex systems and their components are recognisable as a result of difference. Difference is thus a resource to be cherished, not a problem to be solved.

Diversity and discourse

Mogens Sorensen's contribution explored discourse complexity and diversity using compression-based clustering. In this he pointed out that innovations in fields of practice constantly add new aspects to a practitioner's discourse, resulting in a vast, and expanding, abstract event space of realised, unrealised, as well as unrealisable, practices. No single practitioner is able to grasp all combinations of available innovations, and exploration of possibilities thus becomes a matter of local search, bounded by incomplete knowledge and cognitive constraints.

It is common to project multidimensional data to lower-dimensional visualisations for interpretive purposes. With regard to scientific production, bibliometric methods offer explorative and analytical means for visualising patterns in the literature. However, although practitioners, too, share written accounts and scenarios with colleagues, the resulting corpus may be heterogeneous, and omissions of author name, affiliation or references may make it difficult to process such cases by systematic bibliometric means. Alternative methods exist for classifying and visualising heterogeneous information, but in many cases the processing of data is prohibitively labour demanding.

Measuring diversity of a discourse in an abstract sense (understood as diversity against any possible classification scheme) might seem a daunting task, considering the vast number of possible dimensions in discourse. However, progress in bioinformatics and related fields has produced potent methods for exactly this purpose. 'Clustering by compression' [2] is a new method, supported by open-source software, with immediate and practical applications in explorative and analytical complexity research. It is well known that complex texts are less compressible (algorithmically) than simple ones. Along the lines of the Minimum Description Length Principle, what the theory underlying 'clustering by compression' predicts is that if any similarities exist between two texts, they can be algorithmically compressed more efficiently together, than they can apart. Thus, similar texts will co-compress more efficiently, than will dissimilar ones.

The relative difference between the outcome of single and pair wise compression runs can be used to calculate a normalised information distance between two texts. No domain knowledge is necessary, and unsupervised discourse analysis is thus possible.

The information distance matrix, in turn, can be used in hierarchical clustering, multidimensional scaling, or network graphs producing visualisations, which allow the reader to interpret the data in an intuitive manner. Event space thus becomes more a spatial tool than a spatial metaphor. Data clusters, and the distances between and within clusters, may be interpreted as indicators of innovativeness and imitation in the observed field of practice. Changes in data clustering in time sequences of data may be interpreted as trends. Isolated and persistent clusters may be interpreted as stable niches. The method was applied to a sampled corpus of practitioners' self reports of attempts to implement ICT in education. By mapping the texts according to the calculated normalised information distances between them, diversity and complexity within and between samples is assessed and discussed, with regard to the context of regulation.

The problem addressed here is to explore whether it is possible to observe any effects of regulatory interventions or resource competition in the diversity of the discourse over time. Based on the case data, the author discussed whether it is possible to observe sudden shifts in the diversity of the discourse over time.

Biology
Innovation in biology and technology: exaptation precedes adaptation

The importance of diversity in biological evolution was presented by Pierpaolo Andriani and Jack Cohen. They put forward the view that at the root of any adaptive trajectory it is usual for a structure to have been subverted – perverted – to a new function: what Gould and Vrba called 'exaptation'. Generally, this has been regarded as contingent, serendipitous. They believe that 'complexity' rather than reductionist models, particularly plotting the geography of exaptational phase space, suggest several regularities that could be exploited to explain puzzling biological innovations and perhaps to develop a new strategy for technological/industrial innovation. They gave historical examples, including radio tubes (valves), feathers and teeth, as well as cases where biological understanding has enabled technical exaptation. They conclude that the driver of exaptation is not just function and form but context.

Nearly all biological adaptations, and many commercial products now suited to particular markets and functions, began life as something different. The challenge is to understand how the leap to the new function – before the adaptational trajectory that we think we usually understand – can be conceptualised other than as accident, contingency, serendipity. Innovation-by-adaptation, or the *Market-pull* model of innovation, is what traditional business schools teach. We have not taught innovation-by-exaptation because the new connection *creates* the new phase space; it is not that there was an island of possibility waiting to be exploited [3], but that a *new* domain appeared in the universe of possibilities. Can we find the parameters for a phase space of exaptations?

Several classical concepts have changed their usage in ways that help our conceptualisation here. Biological/ecological 'niche' used to refer to some pre-formed – or perhaps Platonic ideal – function waiting for an organism to evolve into it: as in 'The scavenger niche has been emptied now we've killed off the vultures in India; what will replace them in that niche?' In contrast to this lock-and-key image (Odling Smee *et al.* [4]), we have seen a niche as a complicity between a lineage of organisms and the environments it is inhabiting and changing: a creative process, not a habitation-for-rent. This is just the difference between exaptation and adaptation. Because new niches are often repeated during evolution and the parallel innovations are quite detailed, they do seem to be rule-constrained. This is in contrast to the usual belief that they are simply contingent.

Cichlid fishes in Lakes Victoria, Malawi and Tanganyika invented parallel arrays of unlikely specialisations: in the three lakes the different riverine originators diversified into 'species flocks' that included adapted plankton feeders, rock-scrapers and specialised piscivore predators. But all three lakes also have cichlids that have exapted to eating the babies from the mouths of other (mouth-brooding) species, others that specialise in eating only the eyes of other fishes, and some have exapted hinged teeth to scrape off the scales around the tail of a caught-but-not-swallowed prey. All of this requires a jump to a new function and cannot adapt smoothly [5]. But there have been temporal repeats too, as in the sagas of acquisition of sabre-teeth in creodonts and horns in titanotheres. Each drives the other to extinction along an arms-race adaptational trajectory, then the exaptation repeatedly re-arises from the smaller-bodied parent stocks without sabres or horns. These examples strongly suggest contingent but rule-driven innovations. There are parallel innovations, such as the phenomenon of 'steam-engine time' when everyone invented steam engines; in biology, 'natural-selection time' for Spencer, Darwin and Wallace. All these cases suggest that the opportunities for exaptation are at least as much to do with context as with the nature of the tool or the nature of the task. Can we distinguish between rule-driven exaptations and the Conway-Morris adaptational trajectories [6]? We believe his model to believe the intelligent design promoters who maintain the same function throughout an evolutionary event.

What properties of the context are permissive for exaptations? Clearly, a sparse, almost uninhabited region of phase space has few opportunities for the contiguities necessary to establish functional bridges among tools, technologies or indeed species. When sound-recording began, wax cylinders, discs then early wire recorders, as electricity came into technical use; there were few contiguities. Equally, a very crowded region probably fosters high competition, low 'rents' and unacceptable costs for the initial stages of an exaptation, before progression on the adaptational trajectory. The early lake with few fishes gave few if any opportunities; equally, when the ecosystem had matured into hundreds of specialised niches, there was no physiological 'room' to experiment. However, as the era of electrical-recording was paralleled by the digital revolution in electronics, the subversion of digital compact-disc technology to music, and then to sound-and-picture DVDs, was inevitable. Now the music-recording has leapt over into solid memory, and adaptational trajectories involve compression techniques and display/play development. There is a further parameter, though. Silicon Valley has exploded away from the sparse/dense constraint. It is a multidimensional network of reconfiguration experiments. Exposure to new contexts (projects) favours translation of tools into new functions ('horizontal' exaptation), whereas co-optation of tool modules into new architectures ('vertical' exaptation) generates new technological families. The system has became autocatalytic, almost 'mesobiotic'.

In conclusion, enhanced models of evolution, based on a multilevel, hierarchical understanding of biological and technological world, can help the innovation process. In particular, the concepts of horizontal and vertical (or recombinant) exaptation have the potential to provide managers (and policy makers) with an additional tool to increase the speed of innovation processes.

Organic agriculture

In a presentation about organic agriculture, Richard Taylor discussed the relation between diversity and organic farming methods, pointing out that organic growing is associated with much higher levels of agricultural and ecological diversity than conventional farming. It requires a systems-based approach using all beneficial practices and not being selective. As a result of this diversity, organic systems are considerably more sustainable, adaptive, and innovative than traditional ones. These factors could be beneficial in the following ways:

1. Sustainable: as part of a more 'holistic' system of agriculture, organic methods reduce the reliance upon off-farm products such as artificial fertility, biological controls and commercial seed, thus promoting farm independence, food security and more careful management of environmental resources.
2. Adaptive: because organic farms already have a better internal balance and diversity, they are better able to cope with change caused by external factors (for example, new legislation, new technology of production) and they are less vulnerable to 'food scares'.
3. Innovative: as a result of sustainability and adaptive capacity, organic farms and firms are able to be more proactive in developing knowledge-intensive and innovative practices (for example, in defining new standards), leading to a diverse range of new products and opportunities.

Supported by experimental trials dating back 30 years, the logical argument for organic methods is very clear. However, the political will has lagged behind. Only since the 1990s has the development potential been recognised and legislated for by policy makers in government and other institutional agencies. Considering the substantial drivers of change in the modern food industry, namely growers' 'adoption of alternative methods and customers' desires for products and production processes that are health-orientated, environmentally friendly and ethical, the benefits that accrue from diversity in organic/holistic methods can no longer be sidelined.

Standards, certification and labelling are the regulatory instruments that facilitate the development of the sector, and the interplay among these instruments and the social actors that affect and are affected by them, is the subject of this research project.

We presented a case study of Stockfree Organic Services (SOS), a network of organic growers and their associates who are devoted to the promotion of a new 'higher' standard of organic production. SOS uses decentralised systems for processing, distribution and marketing of products, such as farmers' markets and/or box-systems, which operate on a local scale. If the focus upon such local systems of food production and consumption systems can be maintained in a significant way during further adoption of the standard, then there are positive externalities associated with these changes. Improving local self-sufficiency in agriculture can help to rebuild local economies and infrastructure by bringing job security and more equal income distribution to rural areas. Moreover, opportunities for innovation in this sector are currently very strong. The author argues that SOS should be conceptualised as a complex system of culture.

From biology to social systems
Evolution, cognition and identity

Peter Allen and Mark Strathern discussed the importance of micro-diversity in maintaining the richness of natural ecosystems has been established [7–9]. The key answer is that what is missing is the *internal diversity of the populations*. In chemistry, one molecule is very like another, and the only difference is their spatial location. Dissipative structures can create spatio-temporal patterns because of this. The identity of simple molecules is more or less fixed. But the identities of organisms can differ in very many ways. Firstly in location, but also in age, size, strength, speed, colour, etc., and so this means that whenever a population, X, is being decreased by the action of some particular predator or environmental change, then the individuals that are most vulnerable will be the ones that 'go' first. Because of this, the parameter representing the average death rate will actually change its value as the distribution within the population X increases the average 'resistance'. In other words, the whole system of populations has built in through the internal diversities of its populations, a *multiple set of self-regulatory processes that will automatically strengthen the weak, and weaken the strong*. In the same way that reaction diffusion systems in chemistry can create patterns in space and time, so in this more complex system, the dynamics will create patterns in the different dimensions of diversity that the populations inhabit. But neither we, nor the populations concerned, need to know what these dimensions are. It just happens as a result of evolutionary dynamics.

The reason why our 'description' of an ecosystem is not sufficient to understand how it emerged, and what dimensions and factors really play a role in maintaining it, is that any natural ecosystem, or complex economy, really emerges through micro-exploratory processes. As a result, our crude description cannot take into account the real interdependences between different types of agent or individual (Table 3.1). In other words, the description, map or image of something is not the something!

This succession of models arises from making successive, simplifying assumptions, and therefore models on the right are increasingly easy to understand and picture, but increasingly far from reality. *They also are shorn of their capacity for the participating identities to evolve – their real underlying exploratory, error-making processes.* The operation of a mechanical system may be easy to understand, but that simplicity has assumed away the more complex sources of its ability to adapt and change. They become more like 'descriptions' of the system at a particular moment, but do not contain the magic ingredient of micro-diversity that will really allow the

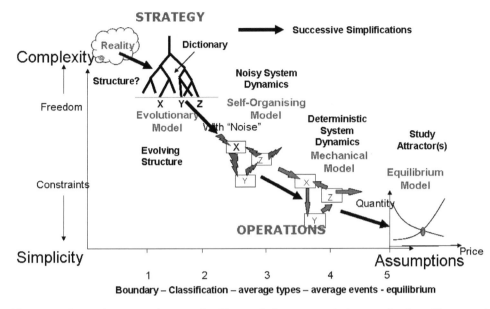

Figure 3.1. Successive assumptions can simplify complexity to successively more simple and less correct representations.

system to undergo structural change and create a new, qualitatively different system, with some new variables and some emergent performance. The ability to adapt and change is still present in the 'evolutionary' model that only makes assumptions 1 and 2, but not those of average type and average behaviours. This therefore tells us that the evolutionary capacity is generated by the behaviours that are averaged by assumptions 3 and 4 – average types and average events – and therefore that organisations or individuals that can adapt and transform themselves do so as a result of the generation of micro-diversity and its interactions with micro-contextualities. This tells us the difference between a reality that is 'becoming' and our simplified understanding of this that is merely 'being' [10].

TABLE 3.1. Interdependences between different types of agent or individual

Number	Assumption made	Resulting model
1	Boundary assumed	Some local sense-making possible: no structure supposed
2	Classification assumed	Open-ended evolutionary models: identities change over time
3	Average types	Probabilistic, nonlinear equations: identities are assumed fixed
4	Average events	Deterministic, mechanical equations: identities are assumed fixed

These ideas are presented in biological populations and then in the evolution of economic markets and organisations.

We can now draw some conclusions concerning the level of 'cognition' required by organisms, individuals, firms/agents to survive in evolving structures. Broadly speaking, we see that almost no knowledge is required for 'agents' to generate successful heterogeneous complexes. Providing that there is micro-diversity among the agents, even with an entirely 'random' basis, eventually the evolutionary system will discover a structure that is stable. In the economic market example, we know that purely random explorations, with no consideration of what seems to work, and what the successful directions seem to be can lead to a very slow rate of improvement of performance. In the further simulations, slightly more sophisticated learning methods are supposed in which either successful competitors are imitated, or trials are conducted to allow 'hill-climbing' behaviour of the profit slope, but all of these require only very limited cognitive power. The 'intelligence' that apparently underlies a coherent market structure lies not within the agents/firms that participate within it, but in the nonlinearities inherent in the economic interactions that are present: the economies of scale, the fixed and variable costs, and the degree of discrimination of potential customers. In reality, collective intelligence is what emerges through evolution and this really requires very little cognitive power on the part of the participating individuals.

In the second example of structural evolution at the level of the internal structure of competing agents/firms, we see that it is the very ignorance of actual consequences of adding one practice rather than another that generates diversity of the different agents/firms, and allows a successful evolution of the industry. The evolutionary models described above show us the importance of the multi-level nature of socio-economic systems. Individuals with characteristic and developing skills and particularities form groups within companies, generating specific capabilities and particular receptivities for possible future changes. The products and services that emerge from this are perceived by a segmented and heterogeneous population of potential consumers, who are attracted by the qualities of a particular product or service and the low price at which it is offered. This results in a market share and in changing volumes of activity for different firms. When volume increases, economies of scale occur and allow further price decreases and greater attractiveness for potential customers. However, debts can be cleared quicker if higher prices are practised, and because there is an interest rate in the model, paying off debt is also a way of reducing costs.

The important result from these multi-agent, complex system simulations discussed above is that instead of showing us *the* optimal strategy for an agent or firm, they tell us that there is no such thing. What will work for a company depends on the strategies being played by the others. The overall lesson is that it is better to be playing in a diverse market ecology than in one involving mainly imitation. So, having a unique identity and product may seem 'risky', but it is better than simply packing into the same strategy as others. Coupled with having an individual product and strategy, it is an advantage to 'learn'. So, exploring the landscape sufficiently to enable 'hill-climbing' in profit space is generally better than not doing it. However, it does not necessarily solve all problems because the pathway 'up-hill' can be blocked by other firms. In this case a more radical exploration is required with the possibility of a 'big jump' in the product and strategy space.

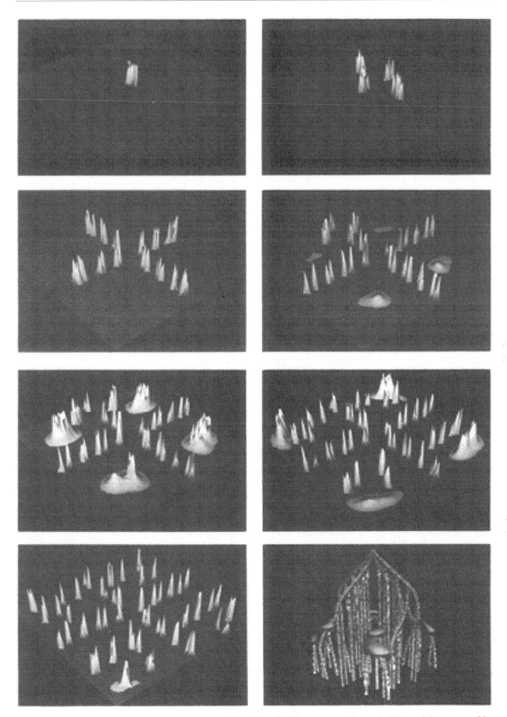

Figure 3.2. In possibility space an initially pure identity will diffuse outwards, and differential success of its heterogeneous populations will provide 'selection'.

The new theoretical framework of evolutionary complex systems is about the emergent and creative co-evolution of identity and diversity at different levels of the system. We have a dialogue between explorations of possible futures at one level, and the unpredictable effects of this both at the level below and the level above. There is a dialogue between the 'trade-offs' or 'nonlinearities' affected inside and outside the particular level of exploration. But it is also true that all levels are exploring. Unless there is an imposition of rigid homogeneity up and down the levels of the system, there will necessarily be behavioural explorations due to internal diversity. In this way, multi-level systems are precisely the structures that can 'shield' the lower levels from instantaneous selection, and allow an exploratory drift to occur, that can generate enough diversity to eventually DISCOVER a new behaviour that will grow. Without the multiple levels, selection would act instantly, and there would be no chance to build up significant deviations from the previous behaviour.

These ideas show us how identities are created and co-evolve in an ongoing evolutionary process, where it is the selection operated by the collective interactions that feeds back on individual experiments. Because of this, we cannot really ever fully understand why things got to be as they are, and in what precise way they may evolve. We cannot understand the multiplicity of micro-events that created the micro-diversity underlying an ecology, an evolving economic market, an evolving organisational form or industry, or a community. It does, however, show us that all these phenomena obey the same generic behaviour – that of evolving complex systems. Individuals and organisations within such systems need to be 'evolvers' if they are to endure over time – to both encourage and allow exploration and to pick up on what works and what doesn't. Instead of fossilising our identity, skills, role or knowledge, we need to keep pushing back its limits, trying new things and learning things even though we cannot say ahead of time what the exact purpose will be. Fortune favours the brave – those that are prepared to move on, to change and to adapt, and because the future is not known then we cannot prescribe the 'best' things to learn. However, by exploring our own diversity and building upon it, we create a richer set of possibilities on which the collective system can thrive, and providing that multiple connections are tried out, then there are multiple possible new synergetic bundles that can emerge. So, the fact of uncertainty about the future leads naturally to a divergent, branching evolution of possible identities and diversities, which then compete and cooperate leading to the selection of compatible subsets, creating multiple possible futures, some of which at least will survive.

Multilevel multidimensional networks for managing complex human systems

In his presentation, Jeff Johnson showed how human systems are characterised by relationships, including interactions between pairs of people, as in a conversation or telephone call, and interaction between sets of people, as in a departmental meeting. Social networks have nodes to represent people and links to represent their pair-wise interactions. The natural generalisation of this is to let a triangle represent the interactions between three people, a tetrahedron represent the interactions between four people, and a multidimensional n-hedron represent the interactions between n people. There are many other kinds of relationship, including those between people and social organisations such as a company or government department. Also, there are relationships between organisations. A particularly important class of relations includes those that assemble people into the social structures we call teams, departments, units, divisions, head office and so on. Another class of relations assembles these substructures into multilevel systems, with multidimensional horizontal and vertical dynamics. Socio-technical systems involve relationships between humans and physical systems, such as business systems, health systems, transportation systems, retail distribution systems, agricultural systems, military systems and many more. This paper will show how the mathematics of multidimensional networks can give a coherent way of representing multilevel human systems and their multidimensional dynamics, including the dynamics of self-organisation, emergence, adaptation and co-evolution between subsystems. In this context it is possible to make well defined the issues of planning and managing such systems, as a step towards a rigorous theory to support effective practice.

Diversity and efficiency: two complementary forces in economic development

Pier Paolo Saviotti described how the diversity of the economic system has increased considerably in the course of economic development and in particular in the period since the Industrial Revolution [11]. The problem can be interesting for economics to the extent that this growth in diversity is not purely a by-product of previous economic development without any implications for future development. In this paper the changing composition of the economic system that a growing diversity entails is considered a determinant of future economic development. The paper will proceed to articulate the reasons for which diversity growth is an important ingredient of economic development and why it is complementary with respect to efficiency growth. To do this a digression on the different types of diversity and on their measurement will be required. Subsequently, a model of economic development by the creation of new sectors will be discussed to provide partial confirmation that diversity growth is a necessary, although not sufficient, condition for long-term economic development. Finally, the relationship of diversity and connectivity will be discussed, both for what concerns material production and the production of knowledge.

Typology and measurements of diversity

Diversity is intended here to refer to the number of *distinguishable* economic species in an economic system [11–13]. Its use needs to be carefully distinguished from that of variety as *dispersion* of measurable properties of economic agents, for example the dispersion of firm productivity within an industry. The concept of diversity as used in this paper refers to the number of distinguishable, and thus qualitatively different, economic species in a system. Each one of these species (for example, a technology with several associated firms) can have a time path during which the dispersion of its measured properties changes systematically. It is better to reserve the term diversity for the use proposed in this paper and to call the other magnitude variance or dispersion (e.g. of productivity). Furthermore, we can distinguish output diversity and process diversity, or focus on the diversity of countries, regions, etc. All these types of diversity have different time paths and interact with one another.

Diversity and efficiency

In this section, two hypotheses about the role of diversity and efficiency in economic development are formulated [11]:

H1. The growth in diversity is a necessary requirement for long-term economic development.

H2. Diversity growth, leading to new sectors, and efficiency growth in pre-existing sectors, are complementary and not independent aspects of economic development.

These hypotheses are justified by the potential imbalance between productivity growth and demand growth in a system at constant composition. Diversity growth provides compensation for the labour and capital saving trend implied by the previous imbalance, while efficiency growth in pre-existing sectors creates the resources required for search activities, leading to the generation of new economic species [14]. In other words, diversity growth can save the system from a trap created by its own previous development.

Economic development and growing diversity

The role of the growth of diversity and its impact on the time path of the economic system will be discussed using a model of economic development by the creation of new sectors. In this model the saturation of a pre-existing sector induces the creation of a new sector [15–17]. Diversity is here measured by the number of sectors in the system. The implications of diversity growth for sustainable long-term growth are discussed. The model shows that under a wide range of conditions the emergence of new sectors and the consequent rise in diversity can give rise to a stable macroeconomic employment growth path, even when each sector tends to create decreasing employment to produce its output. Thus, the model provides partial confirmation for hypothesis H1.

Among the features of the model used in this paper there is the co-evolution of technologies and institutions. In particular, the rate of entry into any new sector is determined by the joint effect of the expected size of the market and by financial availability, which in the paper represents the fraction of the total financial resources allocated to the new sector. The allocation of financial resources to the new sector often requires new competencies, leading to the creation of new institutions, an example of which would be venture capital firms. This is a specific example of the more general situation of the co-evolution of technologies and institutions. If financial resources increase with the size of the output of the new sector, this provides a synergistic effect which raises the rate of growth of the new sector above the average rate of growth of the economy and allows the new sector to achieve its 'economic weight'. The co-evolution of technologies and institutions is also an example of *autocatalysis* [18]: one of the outputs of the process (new firms or a new type of output) accelerates the process itself. Autocatalysis is required in order for a homogeneous system to acquire *structure*.

Diversity and connectivity

The new economic species created by economic development are not independent. They are linked by relationships of input-output, by flows of knowledge, by trade, by regulatory relationships, etc. Thus, they are involved in networks. The structure and dynamics of these networks and their influence on system performance then become very important problems. If diversity grows, we can expect the number of nodes of the global economic network to increase, thus satisfying a necessary condition to be scale free [19–22]. Some socio-economic networks are scale free. However, the dynamics of these networks is as important as their static structure. We can expect new economic species to be poorly connected at the beginning of their life cycle and to develop links both with existing networks and between themselves in the course of time. We can expect the density and the connectivity of the economic system to vary in the course of time, for example falling after the very rapid introduction of new economic species, and rising in periods when not many new economic species are created. For what concerns the effect of these static and dynamic properties on system performance, we can expect a growing density/connectivity to improve the coordination among economic agents and the efficiency of resource utilisation. However, a very efficient but very rigid economic network may not necessarily provide the most favourable conditions for innovation.

In summary, in this section the role of diversity and of efficiency in economic development and their relationship to network density and connectivity will be analysed.

Diversity and interdependence as determinants of network adaptability: qualitative case studies and agent-based modelling

In this section, Manuel Cartier and Ana Colovic described how diversity and interdependence affect the adaptability of a network in the period of major environmental change. They described case studies involving 10 Japanese small-firm networks confronted with the problem of industry relocation to China. The adaptation patterns observed in networks are coherent with the results of Kauffman's [23] NKCS model. A comprehensive reading of the results of the qualitative study through the metaphor of adaptive complex systems [24] enhances our understanding of the network dynamics.

This section addresses the question: How do the characteristics of the structure of a network influence its adaptability? Actually, as Achlor and Kotler note, 'outcomes increasingly are decided by competition between networks of firms rather than competition among firms' [25: p.146]. In particular, the paper examines how diversity and interdependence affect the network's capacity to adapt in the period of major environmental change. This capacity to adapt is considered as an indicator of a competitive advantage, at the network level.

Diversity can be defined as a measure of the variety of living things in a community, based upon one of several mathematical formulae, which account for both numbers of species and numbers of individuals (relative abundance) within species [26]. Now, let us think about diversity at the network level. In a network, we can consider that groups of firms will develop bundles of resources to match each of their client demand. Thus, if we define species as a set of resources associated to one client, we can propose two kinds of diversity:

■ Internal diversity refers to the number and variety of resources used to develop a specific production system. While firms can be considered as bundles of resources [27, 28] by extension, a network too can be seen as a bundle of resources, which is comprised of resources and competences of the network member firms. The structure of this bundle (in particular, in terms of the number and the variety of resources) is the first indicator of the diversity of a network.

■ External diversity refers to the number and variety of clients of the network. Firms depend not only on internal but also on external resources [29], mainly clients.

Interdependence means that actions of an entity have consequences on related entities and system itself. Complex behaviour arises from inter-connectivity of elements within a system and between a system and its environment. That is why two forms of interdependences can be distinguished:

■ Internal co-evolution density refers to different types of ties firms are embedded in. Even though embeddedness in relations is in itself beneficial [30], a too high level of embeddedness has negative effects [31]. Indeed, as loose coupling [32] (Granovetter, 1973) or the existence of structural holes, the non-redundancy relationships [33] are necessary for a system to be flexible.

■ External co-evolution density refers to the interdependence between clients. If clients are competitors, partners, external co-evolution is high.

To understand how diversity affects network dynamics, we conducted a field study in industrial districts in Japan. Several empirical results could be drawn from the study:

1. A mixture of static and dynamic competences in the network enhances its adaptability. Thus, if there are both static and dynamic competences in the network bundle, the reorientation of the network to fit the changing environment seems easier.
2. The diversity of internal ties within a network enhances its adaptability. Networks characterised by the diversity of internal ties (social ties in addition to business ties) seem more adaptable than networks poor in diversified ties.
3. A moderate number of clients enhances adaptability.

The NK model deals more specifically with the interconnections between constituting units of members of the studied system. It is at the origin of one of the most striking results of the complexity theory: the performance is maximal when the level of interconnection between units is neither too strong nor too weak. On the other hand, the NKCS model, which includes the external co-evolution, has been rarely applied to a population of firms [34].

The model NKCS gives the following results:

1. As N and K increases, short-term performance increases: agents are evolving more rapidly. Firms can reach sticking points (configurations of choices from

which they do not move) after a small number of period. 'As K increases, the proportion of agents reaching Nash equilibria increases' [23: p.143].

2. If K is low, a high level of N does not have any impact on performance. Internal diversity within a network is essential for its adaptability. But this diversity performs its role only through internal co-evolution density. Diversity within a network (N) is of no interest unless the internal ties (K) are relatively important. 'Too large a group, and external co-evolutionary density may be diffused' [34: p.306].

3. The ambivalence of internal co-evolution (K) is linked to the trade-off between rapidity of the change and long-term performance, in other words exploration and exploitation. In a network, moderated ties enable a satisfactory adaptation. Too few ties slow down adaptation, while too much ties dam up long-term adaptation.

4. External co-evolution (C) slows down adaptation. Each change of clients pushes the network members to adapt.

5. When NK is sensibly superior to CS, the system adapts rapidly, and then is stable. In a network, the relative weakness of external ties restrains the change of highly linked firms.

6. When NK is sensibly inferior to CS, the system changes rapidly, in a chaotic manner. In a network, the high number of clients creates changes, which destabilise weakly tied networks.

7. The optimal level of adaptability is obtained when NK is close to CS. For Kauffman, 'internal epistatic coupling of each member of a species should be important enough to counterbalance the epistatic coupling between partners' [23: p.280]. In other words, networks have to adjust the ties among their members to the ties between their members with their client. This result generalises the well-known Lawrence and Lorsh [35] differentiation/integration theory.

The authors therefore successfully demonstrated how diversity and interdependence affect network adaptability in a changing environment.

Business ecosystem as a tool for the conceptualisation of the external diversity of an organisation

In their presentation, Mirva Peltoniemi, Elisa Vuori and Harri Laihonen discussed diversity from the viewpoint of an organisation that operates in a business ecosystem. An organisation, as a part of a business ecosystem, makes conscious decisions about its internal structure and aims to adjust its internal diversity to the diversity of its environment that is conceptualised as external diversity in this paper. The ideas presented here do not concentrate on internal diversity of an organisation as such. The focus is on conceptualising the external diversity that is created by the rest of the business ecosystem. External diversity sets the requirements for internal structures and for the internal diversity that are formed by different knowledge domains and different backgrounds of its employees. In this section, concepts such as interconnectedness, competition, co-operation and adaptation are seen as essential factors of the environment and its diversity. The authors argue that in such a co-opetitive environment seeing an organisation as part of a larger system will give useful insights. A business ecosystem as a whole is not able to optimise since the actors do not have all the required information to do so. For this reason an organisation should acknowledge its position as part of a system which requires compromises to be able to make reasonable decisions from the ecosystem's viewpoint. This means avoiding sub-optimal decisions that would hurt the business ecosystem as a whole. The large number of participants that are interconnected have many kinds of interaction, which leads to co-evolution. These interactions may be competitive, co-operative or co-opetitive. The interconnectedness of the organisations also leads to a future that the organisations share at least partly. For example, the success of one organisation may bring success to the other organisations as well. The business ecosystem is located in some environment that consists of many different aspects, such as political, cultural, social and legal. This environment has an impact on the business ecosystem, but the business ecosystem may also have an impact on the environment.

Related to diversity, an organisation seeks the so-called 'sweet spot' of internal diversity. This refers to a beneficial, not optimal, state between excessive disorder (too much diversity) and excessive order (too little diversity). Clippinger claims that 'here on the edge of chaos the system, in this case organisation, is maximally responsive to the variety of its environment but sufficiently structured that it can act and perpetuate itself' [36: p.9].

According to the idea behind the concept of sweet spot, internal structures should be adjusted according to the external variety – the fitness landscape and its diversity. A fitness landscape is a representation of the diversity of the organisation group. If the organisations are clustered in the fitness landscape the diversity of the group is low. On the other hand, if the organisations are scattered on a wide area the diversity of the group is high. Clippinger argues that 'the strategic challenge for management is to characterise accurately the degree of internal and external complexity of an organisation in order to select the appropriate strategy to achieve sustainable fitness' [36: p.26]. Ashby [37] has conceptualised this balance between internal and external diversity with the concept of requisite variety. According to this law, there is no sense of creating complex internal processes if those are not needed, nor is it possible to survive with too simple processes in a complex environment.

The biggest distinction between economic and ecological systems is the ability of people to make conscious decisions, whereas in biological systems there is no conscious intent of that kind. But, according to Hodgson [38: p.197], 'it is widely, but wrongly, assumed that evolutionary processes lead generally in the direction of optimality and efficiency.' According to Hodgson [38: p.201], natural selection leads only to the tolerably fit, not to the superlative fittest. Potts [39] states that selection as a filtering mechanism does not favour the most profitable, but the sufficiently profitable. Selection does not bring the system to single optimal point but to a 'smudge' of tolerable fitness. Kelly [40: p.470] states that only simple machines can be efficient, whereas complex adaptive ones cannot.

A business ecosystem does not optimise. Selection leads only to the tolerably fit, not to the superlative fittest. Organisations operate within the bounds of rationality with the given resources and the existing information. Bounded rationality is associated with 'satisficing' rather than maximising. Thus, an organisation does not optimise its profit, or whatever its goal is, but it 'satisfices' by performing well enough. An evolutionary process of a business ecosystem leads to the selection of a smudge of tolerable fitness because the conscious decisions of bounded rational people and organisations with imperfect information do not allow optimisation.

Axelrod considers the strategic contribution of landscape theory to be its ability to trigger organisations to recognise the factors of fitness and their change [41: p.95]. An organisation, as a part of a business ecosystem, is struggling to survive in its fitness landscape by making conscious decisions based on the understanding that its current capabilities make possible. The concept of fitness landscape brings out two aspects of organisational environment: the first is that success is relative and the second is that a change in environment alters the requirements for a successful actor. The environment consists of other actors, and the possible combinations of success factors define the fitness landscape. No actor can see if it has attained the highest peak in the fitness landscape. Fitness landscape highlights the importance of diversity in a system. The internal diversity contains the seeds of adaptation and survival. The current fitness landscape favours certain features and types of know-how. Trying to optimise in that fitness landscape may destroy other competences or capabilities of an actor, a company or a business ecosystem. Thus, an organisation and as well an ecosystem should foster diversity, not efficiency, to survive in the long run.

As the business ecosystem moves inside the smudge of tolerable fitness, the fitness landscape of an organisation changes. Thus, the environment of an organisation is always dynamic. As the smudge moves in the fitness landscape of the whole business ecosystem, the environment poses changing requirements for the working of the entire ecosystem. When there is substantial diversity in the business ecosystem the smudge is large. However, this leads to poorer efficiency. There is a trade-off between diversity and efficiency. When the smudge, and thus diversity, is large it is easier to fit inside the smudge. This means that an actor that disappears is easy to replace. That augments the robustness of the system. Diversity is an important concept when it comes to the study of groups of organisations.

Inter-connectivity in organisations: conflictual diversity as a measure of evolution

The presentation made by Liz Varga showed how diversity and inter-connectivity are not only related to the sustainability of natural and human systems, but they are the keys to the evolution of these systems. Diversity as embodied in the histories of individuals within the organisation enables innovation and evolution. This diversity is conflictual when individual histories that have little commonality are brought into proximity by purposeful inter-connectivity. If there is more conflictual diversity within an organisation, there is likely to be increased generative potential of novelty and innovation. The more generative potential of novelty there is, the greater the probability for evolution of the organisation to a higher level of emergence. Too much conflictual diversity may result in conflictual chaos, whereby the organisation bifurcates too rapidly inhibiting evolution.

Connectivity and tensions for innovation and the management of radical change: a comparative study

Christen Rose-Andersen set out to explore the fundamentals of radical change and sustainability for communities of practice in their environment. In this effort, three cases have been chosen to illustrate the application of complex systems thinking and cultural-historical activity theory to the management of radical change. This is demonstrated through looking at the necessary interventions for change to enhance the sustainability of a firm, an industry or a society in their wider environment. These complex evolutionary systems of interactions between the affected stakeholders and their skills, the sharing of often contradicting perspectives, the meeting of a diversity of interests and the taking place of collective learning where language becomes an essential mediator in these processes are viewed in this section.

It is shown that it is important to channel the occurring conflicts due to a diversity of interests between actors into rewards of mutual interest and that the assistance of a third party or external expert as an insider in the process of change is often essential.

Emergence principles as applied to urban planning strategies

In this presentation, Sharon Ackerman examined how theories being explored by complexity research can be applied to the domain of urban planning. She presented ideas developed in an urban design competition that used the concept of 'emergent evolution' as the planning strategy for urban regeneration. The designers who engaged in this competition attempted to develop a series of 'emergent agents' that would interact in ways to produce a collectively auto-catalytic urban environment. This approach rejected master planning scenarios in favour of an unpredictable, bottom-up, self-organising environment. The design proposal illustrates how complexity theory can be applied to urban design, and demonstrates possible mechanisms for promoting a self-generating urban environment.

The paper began by outlining traditional urban planning strategies and their limitations, recognising that the Modernist approach to city making has failed to live up to its promise. Many architects and planners question the success of these methods in dealing with the complex realities of city life. Individuals feel alienated amid abstract modernist forms, which lack personal meaning [42, 43]. More disturbingly, highly uniform and segregated environments lack diversity and opportunities for interaction among communities. Neighbourhoods segregated according to housing prices (and therefore income) have led to gated communities, and increased paranoia and distrust. At the same time suburban sprawl has drained once vital city centres, transforming them into dangerous urban wastelands [44].

During recent decades, post-modern thinkers have criticised the city and tried to look for alternatives. Many advocate a formal approach called 'New Urbanism' [45, 46], which attempts to recreate the formal characteristics of the urban fabric found in traditional cities. This approach, however, still relies upon a central planning authority, preconceived outcomes, and top-down organisation and control. The problem with planning, however, appears to lie deeper than form, and the thesis advanced here is that a central reason for the failure of modern planning principles has been its inherently reductionist perspective: a misunderstanding of the nature of the design problem that has led to rigid and inherently dead solutions.

To date there has been little integration of the ideas from complexity theory into the design fields, with a few notable exceptions [47, 48]. But perhaps cities can best be understood as complex adaptive systems. Seen in this light, planners could begin to explore acting as stewards to foster self-organisation, rather than acting as visionaries who create Master Plans. By understanding the principles of self-organisation and adaptation, we can determine what characteristics need to be in place within a system for self-organising behaviour to effectively occur. We can then use this understanding to analyse cities, and determine where such characteristics are absent, thereby inhibiting self-organising and emergent behaviour. This knowledge will in turn guide our strategies for intervening to promote more effective civic renewal and regeneration.

In 2002, the author, working as part of a design team, entered an 'Ideas Competition' sponsored by the city of Winnipeg, entitled 'City Re-Emerging'. The competition was intended to promote growth and renewal in an inner-city area suffering the effects of urban decay. Teams were asked to examine the district, and propose a master planning strategy for the area. The competition guidelines anticipated the development of a Master Plan, anchored around a lead project. Instead, the team opted to design not a plan, but a system for self-generation, which would be allowed to carve out an ideal niche from the urban fabric according to processes of feedback and interaction. Consideration went into thinking about which initial conditions would best foster an adaptable, auto-catalytic environment, and what mechanisms would need to be in place in order to allow a dynamic process of interaction and generation to begin. The design team illustrated a possible emergent 'scenario' that might result from this process of interaction, rather than illustrating a projected final plan, as would generally be the norm. Thus, rather than trying to control outcomes, the team sought to optimise the process whereby self-generation would occur.

Generally speaking, planning exercises describe an outcome. In our case, we could not describe what the outcome of a self-organising urban realm might be, only what characteristics it would display. We proposed that by allowing the agents to act together, and evolution of the system to unfold over time, we would arrive at an environment that settled into viable, fit niches, in a rich varied setting. Complexity theory gives planners the insights with which to generate tools that enable bottom-up urban form, which will, in theory, be better fit to survive in a resilient, adaptive manner, compared with any structures that are artificially imposed from above. Like a successful ecosystem, cities that emerge according to self-organising principles will have the ability to 'strike an internal compromise between maleability and stability' [49: p.73]. They will be resilient in the face of change, yet not so stable that they are unable to adapt to evolving needs.

Reflections

This brief account of the session that took place in September 2005 as part of the Liverpool Complexity Conference cannot do full justice to the many ideas and rich discussions that took place. Clearly, there is a new understanding that individuality, uniqueness and diversity are not simply accidental variation around otherwise more perfect, reasonable average behaviours. Instead, they are recognised as being at the heart of evolution itself, driving it outwards into new dimensions and providing the dynamic stability and adaptability that can keep systems running in a fluctuating environment. Not only is heterogeneity nature's evolved way of dealing with an unknown future, but it has vital importance to social systems, the way that we see ourselves and others, and how we develop and evolve our identities. In this view, exaptation and adaptation are all part of the rich picture of reality, parts that are excluded in our simplistic representations of that reality in terms of systems, structures or organisations at a given time. Time and irreversible change are the founding elements of an understanding of evolution and of diversity.

References

1. Allen P.M., McGlade J.M. Evolutionary drive: the effect of microscopic diversity, error making & noise. *Foundation of Physics* **17** (7): 723–728. 1987.
2. Cilibrasi R., Vitányi M.B. Clustering by compression. *IEEE Transactions on Information Theory* **51** (4): 1523–1545. 2005.
3. Cohen J., Stewart I. *The Collapse of Chaos: Discovering simplicity in a complex world.* London: Viking. 1994.
4. Odling-Smee F.J., Laland K.N., Feldman M.W. *Niche Construction: The neglected process in evolution.* Princeton, New Jersey: Princeton University Press. 2003.
5. Gould J.S. Not necessarily a wing. *Natural History* **94**: 12–25. 1985.
6. Conway-Morris S. *The Crucible of Creation: The Burgess Shale and the rise of animals.* Oxford: Oxford University Press. 1999.
7. Allen P.M. Ecology, thermodynamics and self-organisation. In: *Ecosystem Theory for Biological Oceanography* (eds Ulanowicz and Platt), pp.3–26. *Canadian Bulletin of Fisheries and Aquatic Sciences*, **213**. 1984.
8. Allen P.M. Why the Future is not what it was. *Futures* **22** (6), 555–569. 1990.
9. Allen P.M. The dynamics of knowledge and ignorance: learning the new systems science. In: *Integrative Approaches to Natural and Social Dynamics* (eds M. Matthies, H. Malchow and J. Kriz). Berlin: Springer Verlag. 2001.
10. Prigogine I. *From being to becoming.* New York: W.H. Freeman. 1981.
11. Saviotti P.P. *Technological Evolution, Variety and the Economy.* Aldershot: Edward Elgar. 1996.
12. Stirling A. On the Economics and analysis of Diversity. SPRU electronic working papers series available at: www.sussex.ac.uk/spru/docs/sewps/index.html. 1998.
13. Stirling A. Diverse designs: fostering technological diversity in innovation for sustainability. Presented at 'The role of diversity in social systems and its relation to innovation'. Bologna, Villa Guastavillani, 12–13 July 2004.
14. Pasinetti L.L. *Structural Change and Economic Growth.* Cambridge: Cambridge University Press. 1981.
15. Saviotti P.P., Pyka A. Economic development by the creation of new sectors. *Journal of Evolutionary Economics* **14** (1): 1–35. 2004.
16. Saviotti P.P., Pyka A. Economic development, qualitative change and employment creation. *Structural Change and Economic Dynamics* **15**: 265–287. 2004.
17. Saviotti P.P., Pyka A. Economic development, variety and employment. *Revue Economique.* Special issue on Structural Change and Growth (ed J.L. Gaffard) **55** (6). 2004.
18. Nicolis G., Prigogine I. *Exploring Complexity.* New York: Freeman. 1989.
19. Barabasi A., Reka A. Emergence of scaling in random networks. *Science* **286**: 509–512. 1999.
20. Reka A., Jeong H., Barabasi A. Error and attack tolerance of complex networks. *Nature* **406**: 378–382. 2000.

21. Reka A., Barabasi A. Statistical mechanics of complex networks. *Reviews of Modern Physics* **74**: 47–97. 2002.
22. Barabasi A., Bonabeau E. Scale free networks. *Scientific American*. May: 52–59. 2003.
23. Kauffman S. *The Origins of Order: Self organization and selection in evolution*. Oxford: Oxford University Press. 1993.
24. Anderson P. Complexity theory and organization science. *Organization Science* **10** (3): 216–232. 1999.
25. Achlor R.S., Kotler P. Marketing in the network economy. *Journal of Marketing* **63** (Special Issue): 146–163. 1999.
26. Cunningham W.P., Cunningham M.A., Saigo B.W. *Environmental Science: A Global Concern*, 7th edition. New York: McGraw-Hill Science. 2001.
27. Wernerfelt B. A resource-based view of the firm. *Strategic Management Journal* **5** (2): 171–180. 1984.
28. Barney J.B. Firm resources and sustained competitive advantage. *Journal of Management* **17** (1): 99–120. 1991.
29. Pfeffer J., Salancik G.R. *The External Control of Organizations: A resource dependence perspective*. New York: Harper and Row. 1978.
30. Granovetter M. Economic action and social structure: the problem of embeddedness. *American Journal of Sociology* **91**: 481–510. 1985.
31. Uzzi B. Social structure and competition in interfirm networks: the paradox of embeddedness. *Administrative Science Quarterly* **42** (1): 35–67. 1997.
32. Granovetter M. The strength of weak ties. *American Journal of Sociology* **78**: 1360–1380. 1973.
33. Burt R.S. The social structure of competition. In: *Networks and Organisations: Form and action* (eds N. Nohria and R. Eccles), pp.57–91. Cambridge, MA: Harvard Business School Press. 1992.
34. McKelvey B. Avoiding complexity catastrophe in coevolutionary pockets: strategies for rugged landscapes. *Organization Science* **10** (3): 294–321. 1999.
35. Lawrence P.R., Lorsh J.W. *Organization and Environment: Managing differentiation and integration*. Boston: Harvard Business Press. 1967.
36. Clippinger J.H. III (editor). *Order from the Bottom Up. The Biology of Business – Decoding the Natural Laws of Enterprise*. San Francisco: Jossey-Bass Publishers. 1999.
37. Ashby W.R. *An Introduction to Cybernetics*. London: Chapman & Hall. 1956.
38. Hodgson G.M. *Economics and Evolution: Bringing life back to economics*. Cambridge: Polity Press. 1999.
39. Potts J. *The New Evolutionary Economics: Complexity, competence and adaptive behaviour*. New Horizons in Institutional and Evolutionary Economics. Edward Elgar. 2000.
40. Kelly K. *Out of Control: The new biology of machines*. Social Systems and the Economic World. Cambridge, MA: Perseus Books. 1994.
41. Axelrod R. *The Complexity of Cooperation: Agent-based models of competition and cooperation*. New Jersey: Princeton University Press. 1997.
42. Venturi R. *Complexity and Contradiction in Architecture*. New York: Museum of Modern Art. 1966.
43. Alexander C. *The Timeless Way of Building*. New York: Oxford University Press. 1979.
44. Davis M. *City of Quartz: Excavating the future in Los Angeles*. New York: Vintage Books. 1992.
45. Krier R. *Urban Space*. New York: Rizzoli International Publications. 1979.

46. Duany A., Plater-Zyberk E. *Towns and Town-Making Principles*. New York: Rizzoli International Publications. 1991.
47. Jacobs J. *The Death and Life of Great American Cities*. NewYork: Vintage Books. 1961.
48. Salingaros N. *Principles of Urban Structure*. Amsterdam: Techne Press. 2005.
49. Kauffman S. *At Home in the Universe*. New York: Oxford University Press. 1995.

CHAPTER 4

Education and complexity

Edited by Tamsin Haggis

Introduction

Teachers, researchers, policy makers and educational managers are all very aware of the complexity of educational processes. Many involved in education, however, often find it difficult to find a satisfactory language to describe and explore what they are engaging with, particularly in philosophical, theoretical and research terms. Complexity theory, with its focus on the dynamics of interacting systems, its attention to the specifics of local interactions, and its recognition of de-centred, multi-factorial types of causation, is generating increasing interest in this field.

The earliest work in education that refers directly to complexity and dynamic systems theories appears to emerge in the 1980s in the work of Daiyo Sawada [1] and William Doll [2]. Still earlier, however, researchers such as Lewis Elton [3] were questioning the possibility of cause–effect explanations in educational situations and arguing for many aspects of what would later be explored using complexity. Elton [3], for example, argues that educational research needs to 'attend to interactions' (p.88); to shift its attention 'from events to relations' (p.89), focus on the study of the uniqueness of particular situations, and develop 'a different attitude to time' (p.90).

In the past 10 years or so, a substantial amount of work in this area has been generated in North America. With the exception of William Doll, who is from the University of Louisana, most of this activity has been generated in Canada, very often from the University of Alberta. Researchers such as Brent Davis, Dennis Sumara, Elaine Simmt and Rebecca Luce-Kapler have been exploring ideas from complexity in a range of areas that include classroom management, the curriculum and teacher education. Much of this work has been done in relation to the teaching of mathematics. From a slightly different perspective, Tara Fenwick, also at the University of Alberta, has discussed complexity in relation to theorising in adult education [4].

The Complexity Science and Education Group, to which many of these researchers belong, maintains a website dedicated to complexity in education [5]. This site has a listing of references related to complexity in general, as well as to education, and also contains a link to a new education and complexity journal entitled *Complicity*. The site also hosts the proceedings of the Complexity Science and Educational Research Conference, which has been organised by the Complexity Science and Education Group for a number of years, attracting about 60 (mostly North American) researchers on each occasion.

It would seem, then, that complexity theory is fairly established in the field of education. From one perspective, as the above makes clear, this is true. However, knowledge and use of this work in mainstream education settings outside North America appear to still be limited. In contrast to the North American conference, which was, at least initially, targeted at an invited group of North American researchers, the call for papers for the Liverpool Complexity, Science and Society Conference was circulated to all major educational research organisations in the UK, as well as to research networks in Australia, New Zealand, South Africa and Canada. This resulted in about 40 abstracts, of which 25 were accepted as papers for the conference. Papers came from Hong Kong (×1), The Netherlands (×1), Canada (×8), Israel (×1), South Africa (×1), the USA (×1), Colombia (×1), New Zealand (×1), Australia (×1), Scotland (×3), Ireland (×1) and England (×5). The papers covered the following areas: organisational behaviour (×1), e-learning (×3), mathematics (×7), philosophy/theory (×6), social regeneration (×1), classroom practice (×3; some of these overlap with the mathematics category), multilingual education (×1) and literary studies (×1). There is also a growing body of work in health and social care education [6], though this generated only two papers for this particular conference.

The sections selected for this book explore perspectives on three different philosophical and theoretical aspects of education, all of which have direct implications for educational practice. Deborah Osberg and Gert Biesta focus on the purpose of education and the nature of the curriculum. They argue that prevailing assumptions about knowledge and the curriculum rest upon an idea of education as 'planned enculturation', which is underpinned by a representational understanding of knowledge and meaning. They discuss the possibilities opened up by replacing such understandings with 'emergentist' epistemologies, and explore the implications of seeing both knowledge and human subjectivity as emerging out of participatory action in the world. For them the idea of emergence opens up a way of thinking differently about education as 'structured guidance' (rather than as a tool for planned enculturation).

Tamsin Haggis looks at the contradictions and problems of conceptualising case-study research in this field. She draws attention to the increasing theoretical interest in learning as a phenomenon which is 'situated', specific to context, and characterised by difference. She suggests, however, that this theoretical shift presents an almost insuperable challenge to dominant epistemologies, which are based upon an ontology which sees particularity as being either anecdotal or as an example of larger classes or structures. Using complexity to reframe this underpinning ontology, she argues that a complexity perspective not only provides a rationale for the study of the specific and the particular, but that it suggests an imperative to research educational phenomena from this perspective.

Finally, Rebecca Luce-Kapler and Dennis Sumara explore the nature of consciousness in relation to the study of literature. Starting from a discussion of consciousness as an emergent phenomenon, they look at the potential role of literary study in developing the 'mind-reading' necessary for awareness of self and others in interaction.

Rethinking schooling through the 'logic' of emergence: some thoughts on planned enculturation and educational responsibility

Deborah Osberg and Gert Biesta

People learn many things regardless of whether they are in schools or not. It is therefore safe to say that learning takes place all the time. But is this education? Supporters of some extreme forms of progressive education might argue that it is. But it could also be argued that education is different from unguided learning in that it directs the kind of learning that takes place. In this way education intentionally shapes the subjectivity of those being educated and this is achieved through the curriculum. The curriculum places conditions on learning and any curriculum that does not place such conditions could be considered uneducational. Furthermore, educators who do not manage to create environments (curricula) that are able to direct the subjectivity of those being educated in a particular way must be considered to have failed in their responsibility to educate.

But if education is educational precisely because it shapes the subjectivity of those being educated, then it is impossible to distinguish this conception of education from planned enculturation or training. It would seem, therefore, that if we want to separate the concept of education from that of unguided learning, we are then lumped with a conception of education as planned enculturation. This introduces a problem. The problem is that in contemporary multicultural societies there are ethical and political issues around decisions about which or whose culture people should be trained into through education. Who decides this and on what grounds? As Michael Apple asks, whose knowledge or culture is of most worth [7]? It is precisely in this regard that we believe complexity science can be of help to educators because it shows how it is possible to keep the notion of education as structured guidance without using it as a tool for planned enculturation. How is this possible?

For a start, it is important to remember that the idea of planned enculturation assumes that it is possible to use the educational curriculum to instil knowledge *of* a particular kind of culture. It relies, in other words, on the idea that knowledge being 'transmitted' (by means of the curriculum) reflects or replicates something that already exists (i.e. something that lies 'behind' knowledge itself), which in turn relies on a representational understanding of knowledge and meaning (knowledge 'represents' that which lies 'behind' knowledge). There are, however, strong arguments against representational epistemology that we do not have the space to go into here. Suffice to say contemporary epistemologies (e.g. constructivism, pragmatism, poststructuralism, deconstruction) hold that knowledge and meaning does not represent something that already exists, but 'emerges' as we participate in the world [8] and does not exist except in our participatory actions. We suggest that these epistemologies could be called 'emergentist' epistemologies. Because planned enculturation is tied to representational epistemology, it seems likely that alternative, emergentist epistemologies could 'free' education from the logic of planned enculturation.

Although many attempts have been made to rethink schooling in terms of emergentist epistemologies, we would argue that all these attempts fail to 'overcome' representational epistemology because they leave intact the idea that the function of schooling is to replicate *in* the learner knowledge *of* some pre-conceived 'way of being'. Gregory Ulmer, for example [9], proposes a 'pedagogy of invention', which he claims is organised around an emergentist epistemology because it suggests that the purpose of a pedagogical presentation or 'performance' is not to transfer a message or replicate the meaning of the presentation in the receiver, but to provoke the receiver to respond to the presentation and so bring forth a wider reading of the presentation itself. For Ulmer, the pedagogical presentation should *generate* rather than *transmit* meaning. It is in this sense that Ulmer's 'pedagogy of invention' makes use of an emergentist epistemology (i.e. meaning 'emerges' from the pedagogical presentation), but this does *not* mean his pedagogy is freed from the logic of planned enculturation. This is evident in the following remark:

> '[a pedagogy of invention is] *intended not only to show people the principles of creativity and how to put them into practice but also … to stimulate the desire to create (not necessarily in 'art' but in the lived, sociopolitical world)*' [9: p.264].

Ulmer, in other words, wants to use the curriculum to *transmit* the 'principles of creativity'. He wants to produce people who are creative, but in doing this he is still channelling the human subject in a pre-determined direction, which means his pedagogy is still a form of planned enculturation.

At this point we could give up and say that it is not possible to free education from the logic of planned enculturation because being an educator is precisely about directing the subjectivity of others towards some cultural end ('way of being'). To give up the attempt to direct the subjectivity of others is to give up education, which would mean there is no way for an emergentist conception of meaning to manifest in an educational context. But we believe there is another way out [10], and it lies in applying the idea of emergence not only to knowledge but to human subjectivity itself. We need a conception of human subjectivity that leaves open the question of what it means to be a human subject. When we no longer assume we know what we are starting with, then there is no way to work out a course of action that causes what we are starting with to end up where we want it to be. This means we can no longer implement a programme of planned enculturation. But how do we leave open the question of what it means to be a human subject? How do we move from a representational conception of human subjectivity, which understands the human subject in terms of *what* it is, to an emergentist conception, which leaves open the question of what it means to be a human subject?

One theorist whose understanding of human subjectivity could be called an emergentist understanding is Hannah Arendt. Arendt frames human subjectivity in terms of 'beginning something new' [11: p.157]. For Arendt, when we begin something we 'show ourselves' in the human world as we do when we are born. In other words, as human subjects we are constantly being 'born' in interaction with others. However, the subjectivity that we reveal through our beginnings is never purely our own because our beginnings are always constrained and therefore 'contaminated' or 'frustrated' by the beginnings of others who are different from us. We are therefore never the sole author or producer of the subjectivity that we 'reveal' through our beginnings. Furthermore, because none of us lives with the same set of others (whose own beginnings 'contaminate' and 'frustrate' ours), this understanding of subjectivity suggests that being with others who are different from us – who 'contaminate' and 'frustrate' our actions – is the only condition in which we can show ourselves in our uniqueness. With this understanding we can begin to understand human subjectivity not in terms of *what* it is, but in terms of *where* the human subject emerges (it 'emerges' *as* it participates in the world and does not exist *except* in its participatory actions) or, in Jean-Luc Nancy's words, 'comes into presence' [12]. According to Nancy this 'coming into presence' is always a unique event, something that 'takes place', and so the subject that comes into presence is always unique, a singular 'who' rather than a case of something more general. We could therefore say that an emergentist understanding of human subjectivity is concerned not with *what* a human subject is but with *who* it is *in interaction with others who are different*.

When we try to understand people in terms of *who* they are in interaction with others, rather than *what* they are, we no longer have a clear starting point or foundation for curriculum theorising and planning because we can never know who we are dealing with. This is because the 'who' that we are dealing with only emerges in our interaction with them, not before or after. For the same reason we can no longer plan a curriculum that aims at some cultural ideal determined in advance. But the loss of a starting point or foundation for the curriculum does not mean that the notion of curriculum is unimportant or that we can no longer theorise about education. It means, rather, that we must theorise education as a trajectory *without* foundations [13]. If human subjectivity emerges in a space of radical contingency – which is a space in which the notion of foundations has no place – then this space is still a *curricular* space, and so it is still possible to theorise education *as* the (foundationless) space in which the human subject emerges or 'comes into presence' [10: p.33]. This space could be called a 'space of emergence'.

The first thing to notice about the curriculum as a 'space of emergence' is that it is not a space of common ground. Because human subjectivity emerges only when one acts with others who are different and who constrain our beginnings [11, 13], this means education only takes place where 'otherness' – being with others who are different from us – creates such a space. Educators therefore have a responsibility 'to make sure there are at least opportunities within education to meet and encounter who and what is different, strange and other' [10: p.69].

Another consequence of understanding education as taking place in a 'space of emergence' is that it becomes necessary to acknowledge that situations in which we are constrained by the beginnings of others, such that it is difficult or impossible to become the 'master of our own actions', are the very situations which are conducive to the emergence of human subjectivity. The educator is therefore responsible *for making education difficult*, for facing people with difficult and uncomfortable challenges that unsettle the doings and understandings of those being educated [10: p.92]. This is contrary to conventional educational logic where it is believed necessary to simplify rather than complicate educational content to aid the understanding of those being educated: help them become the 'master of their own actions'.

Lastly, if educators are responsible for maintaining a space of emergence, then this implies they are *not* responsible for socialising people into a common way of life, but rather for allowing people to emerge as singular and unique beings [10: p.70]. This is very different from conventional understandings of education where the purpose of the curriculum has been to 'iron-out' any idiosyncrasies, so that those being educated can develop in the 'right' way. Conventional school curricula are generally designed with some predetermined (and testable) end in mind. For this reason it could be argued that their objective is to make people part of a system, the structure of which is decided in advance, so that when one part of that system wears out it can be replaced by another just like it. In this sense the purpose of conventional curricula is to produce similar and interchangeable units. But if we hold that education is about the emergence of human subjectivity then such curricula must be seen as un-educational. We do not mean to suggest that there is no place for training. Only we could perhaps distinguish it from 'education'. Our concept of education – unlike traditional concepts that try to use education to produce interchangeable units – is about people being able to emerge as irreplaceable beings, each able to make a unique contribution. Education, in other words, is about the invention or renewal of culture, rather than the replication of a particular cultural ideal.

What we have tried to argue here is that with the concept of emergence it becomes possible to distinguish educational practices from unguided learning on the one hand, where no attempt is made to direct the subjectivity of those doing the learning, and from planned enculturation on the other, where an attempt is made to channel people into a specific culture or way of life. Because both unguided learning and planned enculturation are problematic from an educational perspective, it would seem that the concept of emergence has an important contribution to make to educational theory and practice.

Conceptualising the case in adult and higher-education research: a dynamic systems view
Tamsin Haggis

In terms of the framing and focus of research, recent years have seen a theoretical shift in many areas of the social sciences towards recognition of some of the limits of currently dominant epistemologies. 'Recognising limits' is not meant here only in the sense that there will always be limits to the results of all processes of abstraction aimed at explanation. In addition, research is dominated by particular types of abstraction and explanation, when other types may also be possible.

One aspect of this theoretical shift is an increasing concern with the problems of understanding the local and the specific, and many related issues connected with the particularities of context. Although it can be seen in many different fields in relation to theory, however, the implications of this move have yet to be satisfactorily worked out. In particular, the implications for the analysis of data, and for the epistemologies and ontologies that underpin the analysis of data, have not received a lot of attention (though see [14] and [15]).

Although some researchers may no longer be interested in defining variables, or measuring and counting in relation to large samples, the analytical strategies that are used for more qualitative data (interview narratives, for example) are nonetheless arguably often informed by the same ontological assumptions that underpin the epistemologies that these approaches usually intend to reject. For example, it is largely taken for granted that comparative analysis, in relation to something like interview data, should be performed cross-sectionally, and that the overall purpose of the analysis is the creation of patterns or themes that can be seen to be *common* to the different narratives being examined. But what does a common pattern across different narratives indicate? And how can a pattern that relates to only one particular case be of any use in understanding others?

These familiar questions arise at least partly out of the assumption that it is possible to relate the results of a particular study to other, similar situations, and to form these relationships in quite specific ways. Although this makes logical sense for some of the purposes of research, existing assumptions about the *nature* of this relating are not often examined[1]. The assumption that one situation can or should relate to another is often based upon a belief that the phenomena in question are 'underpinned' by structures and causal factors that the researcher is in some way able to apprehend, or at least speculate upon, from their particular vantage point:

> 'As Ely et al. (1997) describe, qualitative analysis and interpretation of data is similar to climbing a mountain. One gradually achieves a broader view of the data which is likely to be wider than that of the participants themselves' [16].

Qualitative researchers are usually careful to recognise that generalisations cannot be made from small studies. However, the demand to 'draw out' particular types of implication from case studies rests upon a belief in the possibility of something very similar to generalisation, and upon the assumption that what manifests as variety and diversity can be described in terms of subtle forms of 'deep' structure (whether such structures are conceptualised as real, or simply as analytical constructs). An example of this is Goodwin's [17] study of adult learners at university, which identifies three categories of individual: 'pleasers', 'searchers' and 'sceptics'. Transcendent categories such as these function to create an apparent underpinning unity to particular aspects of the different narratives which have been analysed, even though these narratives have been generated from within the very *different* contextual settings of individual people's lives.

Complexity and the conceptualisation of the case

As a set of ideas about process and formation, complexity and dynamic systems theories appear to offer the potential for thinking differently about some of the assumptions inherent in both explanatory and interpretive approaches, and about some the problems these assumptions can give rise to. Although the complexity of the social world, taken as a whole, could be conceptualised as being characterised by 'millions or billions of variables that can only be approached by the methods of statistical mechanics and probability theory' (Weaver, 1948, in Johnson [18]), social complexity could also be conceptualised as consisting of many smaller, overlapping types of organised, but open, dynamic system. Cultures, discourses, social groups, institutions, disciplines and even individuals could all be seen as open systems which manifest different types of organisation through time, in the sense outlined by complexity theory (Figure 4.1).

---

1 Post-modern, post-structural and feminist approaches have done major creative and destabilising work in relation to these assumptions, but the implications of such destabilisation are not frequently carried through to the actual analysis of data.

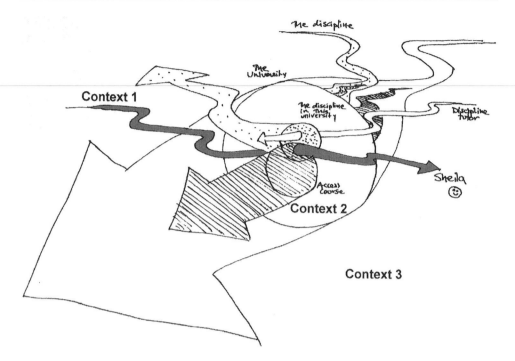

Figure 4.1. Open systems which manifest different types of organisation.

Themes, variables, key factors (deep structures, generalisation)

In anything conceptualised as a complex, dynamic system, the interactions are *multiple*, and *multiply connected*, and it is the multiplicity of the interactions through *time* which produces effects. Causality in this situation therefore, from one point of view, cannot be meaningfully reduced to single or limited numbers of factors or variables, as the factors are all crucially implicated in relation to each other, and change their effects through time. From a complexity perspective, the interactions are not 'underpinned' by any kind of centralised, generative force or structure which could be said to determine their nature; and the idea of emergence in particular confounds this type of deterministic thinking. Though emergence takes place within constraints, such constraints are not the deep structures of a clearly bounded phenomenon. In this situation, Byrne [19] has suggested that the impossibility of tracking multiple interaction histories means that research needs to shift from a focus on *cause* to a focus on *effects*.

Conventional categorising approaches to the analysis of data try to identify structures of meaning which are grounded in individual responses or accounts, but which at the same time in some way also transcend these individual accounts, and thus have the potential to 'illuminate' other manifestations of 'the same type' of phenomena. Complexity, on the other hand, provides a rationale for trying to understand something[2] about how multiplicities of different variables might be

---

2 Importantly, not everything.

interacting *together*, dynamically, to produce particular forms of emergent result. In this situation, the search for causes has, in some important ways, to be abandoned.

The inability to identify centralised mechanisms or to infer causal pathways, however, does not mean that relationships cannot be observed between particular sets of interacting variables (what Goldstein [20] talks about as *conditions* for emergence) and what it is that actually emerges from these interactions (Byrne's *effects*, as above). For example, it could be observed that in the case of a particular institution, with specific types of staff, specific types of curriculum, a particular kind of culture and ethos, and students from predominately x and y type of social backgrounds, particular types of result emerge from the interactions of these different things (think of Oxford University, for example). The absence of a central driver in this conceptualisation suggests a potentially fruitful shift from the search for generic causes (or correlations) towards a closer study of *what* is interacting, over time, and *how* such interactions may be taking place, in relation to the outcomes that can be observed in a specific situation. Though the causal pathways cannot be identified, aspects of the conditions that give rise to particular types of emergence can.

This direction in thinking, however, leads to a focus on particularity that jars with normal expectations which say that a specific case has, in some sense, to be an example of a broader class, or at least an example of how larger structural forces may 'play out' in a particular situation[3]. From a complexity point of view, the dynamic system being studied (for example, a particular institution), while both constrained and also partly constituted by the interactions of other, overlapping systems[4], cannot be conceived of as an example of a type of structure or system, because in some crucially important ways, it will also always be unique. It is not an example of anything; it is itself. This does not mean that no similarities can be observed between this dynamic system and other, related types of system. But thinking of something as a dynamic system provides a rationale for understanding what emerges uniquely from the interactions of that particular system, which is different to the attempt to create categories of similarity which aim to transcend such individual particularities.

Cross-sectional analysis: the problem of understanding difference and local contexts

Because of this connected, multi-factor causality, elements that are isolated and conceptually removed from a system of connected interactions (as a 'theme' may be identified in relation to an individual narrative, or a 'characteristic' in relation to an individual school) in effect cease to have meaning in terms of understanding the system from which they were extracted (although they might have meaning in relation to other such isolated elements abstracted from other systems). To understand the nature, or generation, of what has been categorised as a theme or characteristic, it is necessary (from a complexity perspective) to study the smaller system itself (the individual or school), and to study this in terms of its interactions

---

3 What currently dominant ways of thinking say little about, however, is why such forces play out in a particular way in one example, and in quite a different way somewhere else.

4 Any system could be seen as having particular interaction characteristics, though these would not be 'characteristics' in a fixed or essential sense. In the case of larger social and cultural systems, such characteristics could be something like patterns of class or gender relations.

through time. This places the researcher/educator, conceptually, *within* the system being studied, looking at histories and local interactions, rather than trying to climb Ridley's [16] mountain to get a 'broader view of the data'. Importantly, such a shift also makes the researcher part of the interactions that are being studied, distinguishing a complexity standpoint from phenomenological approaches (which are premised on the assumption that it is possible to 'bracket out' the researcher's part in the research).

Some of these ideas inevitably lead to questions about how systems are to be framed (and by whom), and to questions about how such systems might be understood in relation to each other. This is particularly relevant to the current interest in understanding phenomena as 'situated', or 'in context', and the many problems associated with defining and handling the specificities implied by such interests. Although case studies, for example, can appear to 'study things in context', context seems often to be vague and problematic, not only in terms of how specificity is supposed to link up to generality, but also in relation to how it is conceptualised in relation to: (a) the boundaries of a case; and (b) the relation of the bounded case to the contexts of the individual sub-units within it.

If the intention in an interview-based case study, for example, is to 'interpret meanings in context', then comparative analysis of different interview narratives from a particular context (e.g. a group of access students, an adult education class, etc.) appears to make this possible. However, any 'meanings' that come out of the interview transcripts do not so much relate to the group or class that has been defined as the case, but rather to the local contexts inhabited by the different individuals who have been interviewed. In terms of generative forces, it is arguably these individual contexts (which include but also go beyond the membership of the defined group or class) that have created whatever meanings can be claimed to be expressed in the narratives.

The theme, or group of themes, that might be created in a comparative analysis of different interview texts generated within a case arguably says more about the context/group which has been defined as the case[5] than it does about the individuals within the group. Paradoxically, however (given that individual contexts are not considered in the analysis), the theme is far more likely to be presented as information about the individuals as some kind of type (e.g. 'these adults are all motivated by career prospects') rather than in terms of the context of the case (e.g. 'this university setting, in the context of current political and cultural agendas, encourages these adults to talk about learning in terms of career prospects'). The transcendent category that is the individual type appears to point towards a subtle form of deep structure underpinning the manifest variety of individuals. This type of transcendent category is not problematic as long as it is clearly referring to the dynamic system that has been bounded as the case, rather than the individuals within the case. But if the researcher is trying to understand individual experience, to 'give voice' to individual perspectives, then a comparative analysis of interview texts seems to contradict this intention.

Thinking of people and social/institutional/cultural contexts as complex, dynamic systems allows for the separation of at least three distinct types of context: (1) the contexts of the wider lives and histories of those being interviewed within the

---

5 And, of course, about the conceptual frame of the researcher.

case; (2) the context of the case; and (3) the dynamic systems of culture and society within which the case is embedded. Anything that can be legitimately bounded as a dynamic system[6] will have particular initial conditions, specific interaction histories, and will be interacting dynamically with specific and multiple 'presents', so that in any case study there will be *specific* manifestations of each of these (and other) types of context. Conceptualising these different types of context as dynamic systems allows the researcher to think about conditions and effects relating to the individual histories and current conditions of each different type of context, while at the same time recognising that all of these systems are implicated in each other, in terms of currently manifesting interactions.

Complexity and dynamic systems theories not only provide a rationale for studying the concrete and particular, but, by suggesting that knowledge *can only be* contextual [21], such theories arguably provide an imperative to think about phenomena in this way. While the focus on particularity suggests a departure from currently dominant ontologies, this perspective does not rule out the usefulness of comparative analyses. Complexity, rather, opens up new questions about what can validly be compared cross-sectionally, by framing the focus of research in terms of interactions, conditions and emergent effects. It also opens up thinking about other kinds of comparison (longitudinal, for example, as opposed to cross-sectional). For further exploration of these issues in relation to a study using this conceptual framework in relation to a study into adult learning in higher education, see Haggis [22, 23].

Educating awareness through literary experiences: understanding consciousness as an emergent phenomenon

Rebecca Luce-Kapler, Dennis Sumara and Tammy Iftody

Within the field of consciousness studies, an ongoing debate is occurring about whether 'consciousness' or 'conscious awareness' of self-identity emerges through language or through sensory perception. Neuropsychologist Merlin Donald [24] argues that human consciousness cannot be reduced to either of these. He suggests that the human ability to be perceptually aware of contexts and to notice temporal and other relationships is made possible by the 'hybrid' minds of human beings. That is, while cognitive processes are brain-based activities, the development of them depends upon networked representation and storage systems that exist outside the individual human biological body. From this perspective, identity is paradoxically both private and public. As Donald explains, the 'ultimate irony of human existence is that we are supreme individualists, whose individualism depends almost entirely on culture for its realisation' [24: p.12].

---

6 Discussion of this is beyond the scope of this section. From one point of view, what is bounded as a dynamic system is the creation of the researcher, underscoring the point that from this perspective the researcher is conceptualised as being an integral part of the study in a way that is not recognised by many other epistemological approaches. However, most discussions of dynamic systems do provide certain criteria that would have to be met in terms of a definition (see, for example, Cillers, 1998); only certain types of phenomenon could be described in this way.

Although human beings are continually interacting with their immediate contexts and contacts, most of these interactions remain at a non-conscious level, with consciousness primarily being devoted to the integration of new information. This is not a new insight. Nearly a half-century ago, Merleau-Ponty [25] argued that most of human consciousness is preoccupied with creating bridges between memory and projections of the future. Curiously, then, one's consciousness of self in the present moment emerges not so much from what is presently experienced but, rather, from the interpreted relationships between the remembered past and the projected future. In a strange way, consciousness has no real present time but rather exists in what Edelman [26] calls 'the remembered present.'

This formulation helps us to understand why consciousness has been such a difficult subject for philosophers and for scientists. For although human beings have an *experience* of primary and higher order consciousness, these experiences cannot really be located in any one particular place in the brain. Instead, consciousness seems to be an emergent phenomenon – one that relies on networked relationships between the biological and the cultural worlds. Although conscious experience depends on primary sensory perception and on the brain to process these relationships into language and memory, these abilities are not controlled by any central processor. Instead, they are distributed in neural nets in the brain, which are linked to the nervous system and to the physical world. Furthermore, for conscious awareness (primary order) to become personalised into a sense of self-identity (higher order), an increasingly sophisticated Theory of Mind (mindreading ability) is required to interpret experience.

Emerging around age four, mindreading (also called Theory of Mind) is the innate ability to observe, understand and predict the behaviour of others. This ability allows the child to realise that others have interpretations of the world that may be different from her or his own. Furthermore, this genetic aptitude for building theories of others' minds is constantly being updated and adjusted on-the-fly in response to increasingly complex social interactions. Eventually, the web of social feedback and patterns of response shape a psychology of mind that not only influences the way we interact with others, but also the way we come to experience a sense of self during those interactions. Therefore, the importance of mindreading within social contexts cannot be overemphasised. As Donald argues, 'Human social games are too intricate, unpredictable, and, above all, treacherous to play them on automatic pilot' [24: p.61].

Mindreading is closely linked with the ability to empathise with others and to make ethical decisions emerging from these empathic understandings. As developed by philosopher Evan Thompson [27], recent neurophenomenological research has provided evidence of the biological substrate for mindreading capacity. Most fascinating is research that has documented the existence and function of 'mirror neurons'. Although it is well-established that cognitive processing depends upon the development of complex 'neural nets' that emerge from embodied action, it is now known that it is possible to achieve similar neural-net development through the *observation* of another completing an act – or through the embodied *simulation* of acts. For example, watching another person who is laughing or crying can sponsor neuronal responses that are considered identical to one's own embodied experience of laughing or crying [28]. Although the research is still inconclusive, it is theorised that direct observation may not be necessary for mirror neurons to become enacted:

imaginative visualising, particularly if these generate emotional sensations and responses, are believed to also activate mirror neurons to become organised into neural nets that can influence future behaviour [29]. One could hypothesise, then, that the act of *imagining* identifications with characters is influential to the developing of the neural nets believed to structure human consciousness.

In theorising human consciousness, it is important to understand the fundamental difference between human consciousness and that of other animal species. Although it is certainly the case that most animals have primary consciousness, only human beings have the ability to use narrative and literacy practices to extend the temporal zone of consciousness. The development of narrative forms of language that enable human beings to represent their past, present and projected experiences has allowed us to extend the temporal zone of consciousness from seconds (with gesture) to minutes (with speech). And the ability to be able to represent experience symbolically though alphabetic and analogical forms has meant that the products of consciousness can extend over years and centuries. This is a uniquely human ability. Although higher-order mammals can extend the physiological capacity of consciousness with rudimentary forms of collective cognition and can even generate local 'knowledge', they are not able to 'pass' this knowledge from one generation to another except through copying/mimicking. Human beings, however, can create a 'body of knowledge' that transcends the biological bodies that created it, and thus can both maintain culture and be aware of how culture has changed over generations. Literary fiction and the experiences of consciousness that these support can be considered one important artefact that human beings have developed to extend both the social and cultural temporal zones of conscious awareness.

Literature and the phenomenology of consciousness

Novelist and literary theorist David Lodge [30] argues that the literary novel is an example of a cultural artefact that authors have developed over recent centuries to represent the complexity of human consciousness. Lodge suggests that for engagement with a novel to be relevant to the reader, she or he must be able to discern the consciousness of characters to be able to develop literary identifications with them. It could be argued that the writing and reading of literary novels is an important cultural 'mindreading' practice that helps both writers and readers to better understand how their own consciousness is created, how it functions, and how it evolves over time. What the literary novel can offer beyond what is experienced in other ways by human subjects are opportunities for individual readers to revisit the same text over time and, therefore, to better notice the continued development and evolution of their own sense of consciousness in relation to the consciousness represented by the text.

We offer the following literary texts as illustrative of how literature represents consciousness. Consider a moment in *Mrs. Dalloway*, Virginia Woolf's study of an individual consciousness. The reader lingers in the mind of Clarissa Dalloway during an entire and somewhat memorable day in her life. As she is preparing for a party that is to cap the day, Clarissa looks into the mirror and has a brief moment of insight:

> *'How many million times she had seen her face, and always with the same imperceptible contraction! She pursed her lips when she looked in the glass. It was to give her face point. That was her self-pointed; dartlike; definite. That was her self when some effort, some call on her to be her self, drew the parts together, she alone knew how different, how incompatible and composed so for the world only into one centre, one diamond, one woman who sat in her drawing-room and made a meeting-point ... '*[31].

Just before this passage, Clarissa has had a moment of disquiet about turning 52 and comes to her dressing table to reassure herself and to 'collect the whole of her at one point'. As she gazes into the looking glass, the reconciliation of her self-awareness requires a sharpening or tightening of her efforts and appearance. Clarissa's sense of consciousness requires precision, composure and centeredness.

While Woolf's novel is a fascinating exploration of the fragmentation beneath the more collected narratives of self and an outward composure, Michael Cunningham's novel *The Hours* adds a level of imaginative intertextuality to Woolf's conception of consciousness. In this particular passage, Cunningham steps inside the mind of Virginia Woolf herself, creating the inner monologue as she prepares to write *Mrs. Dalloway*. He imagines the consciousness of the writer imagining the consciousness of a character:

> *'She can feel it inside her, an all but indescribable second self, or rather a parallel, purer self. If she were religious, she would call it the soul. It is more than the sum of her intellect and her emotions, more than the sum of her experiences, though it runs like the veins of brilliant metal through all three. It is an inner faculty that recognizes the animating mysteries of the world because it is made up of the same substance, and when she is very fortunate she is able to write directly through that faculty'*[32].

The result is a different depiction of consciousness from that of Clarissa Dalloway.

Through the persona of Virginia Woolf, Cunningham describes an experience of consciousness that also entails an impending sense of union, but it is not 'pointed' or 'dart-like' like Mrs Dalloway's. Rather it flows, fractal-like and brilliant through all that she is. Much more than the sum of her parts, this 'inner faculty' is attuned to the 'animating mysteries of the world' seeking out the novelty in her experiences. This emergent sense of consciousness as more than the sum of its parts is oriented towards possibility rather than precision. Such a mindset reflects an emergent understanding of consciousness.

Emerging implications for education

We defined consciousness as a symbiotic product of biology and culture. The human 'mind' exists somewhat ambiguously among human brains, other human biological systems and all both human made culture and the more-than-human world. Human consciousness, defined both as perceptual awareness and the experience of knowing that one has awareness (or what we could call experiences of having a 'self') are not 'caused' by neuronal responses to the environment, nor are they caused by the environment itself. Instead, consciousness is a doubly embodied experience that co-emerges with both the biological and the phenomenological.

One primary way that human beings develop self-awareness of their own minds is by becoming aware of other minds. Paradoxically, it is only once we begin speculating on the mental lives of others that we begin to appreciate our own. These 'mindreading' abilities become fundamental to the continual adaptations that human beings must make in their daily lives. We argue that literary experiences create productive mindreading practices that contribute to the ongoing development of the human sense of self-consciousness.

Nevertheless, as we have shown elsewhere [33, 34] that for mindreading opportunities to become maximised, readers need to become aware of their own mindreading practices. In other words, the process by which their own consciousness develops and evolves through literary identifications must become made explicit. One way that this can be done is for readers to notice how authors use textual forms to create the 'minds' of characters. To do this, readers need to become aware of the literary techniques authors use to invent consciousness for characters, and other literary/textual devices they develop to create inter-character relationships within texts.

The now-common reflective response practices that are used in school contexts in North America support a very superficial attention to these concerns. Although students may be invited to explore personal connections to the characters, situations, and so forth, these connections more often serve to confirm already-held beliefs about human nature. However, our recent research has shown that deep understanding of how the 'imagined' and the 'remembered' aspects of human cognition are intimately entwined requires fine-grained critical reading practices, supported by informed discussion and critical reflection [34]. Although some students are intuitively aware of these relationships, most require direct instruction to learn how to notice the deeper structures of literary forms and how these function to support the ongoing creation of conscious awareness. It is through these critical close-reading and other deliberate mindreading practices that readers develop a more sophisticated understanding of the complex ways consciousness emerges from the alliance between cultural forms, memory and currently experienced perceptual awareness.

Our research has suggested that teachers can enhance the complexity of the pedagogical situation to avoid the mere transfer of inert knowledge and reproductive ways of knowing. It has been our experience that many students (especially good readers) often use the text to confirm rather than to question their own beliefs, including beliefs about their self-identity. Teachers need to interrupt the familiar superficial reading practices of students. This requires a kind of mindful attention to the possibilities represented by the text. We argue that superficial readings need to be replaced with close readings that are supported by pedagogical attention to how the literary form is structured and, importantly, how readers become implicated in those forms. Also, readers need to notice how they interpolate the text with their own memories and imaginings and, in so doing, create new literary forms *and* new editions of self-consciousness.

We have found that one way to help readers to notice these complexly nested structures is to ask students to engage in practices of mimicking and copying the forms that they are studying. Good old-fashioned memorising of passages and of transposing representations of personal experience onto existing literary plot structures helps readers to develop a more fine-grained understanding of how the 'minds' of literary characters are created by authors. Experimenting with writing in different genres such as hypertext introduces readers to the techniques of representing consciousness. By engaging in these 'copying' practices, readers not only notice how form influences perception but also how perception influences form.

As well, we have found that teachers must help students to understand that all reading requires a certain amount of 'writing' by readers. However, some texts demand more of this than others. To maximise the developing of self-consciousness, readers need to develop a body of skills that allow them to engage at many levels with a text and with a variety of different texts. In so doing, readers are not merely expanding what they know; they are also expanding and transforming their own sense of consciousness.

Like all complex emergent forms, the experience of consciousness is the product of simple processes, ones that can be noticed and nurtured in the context of the classroom. For teachers of literary texts this means creating enabling constraints [35] that help students become aware of how self-consciousness does not precede or follow pedagogical encounters, but instead emerges from the complexly nested inter-twinings of memory, imagination and sensation. In maintaining an ongoing, coherent sense of self, each of us is required to adjust personal memory with current and projected relationships, contexts and situations. Rendering the bio-cultural hybrid nature of human consciousness visible through literary experience is one way to make such self-conscious practices more deliberate.

References

1. Sawada D., Caley M.T. Dissapative structures: new metaphors for becoming in education. *Educational Researcher* **14** (3): 13–19. 1985.
2. Doll Jr W.E. Complexity in the classroom. *Educational Leadership* **47** (1): 65–70. 1989.
3. Elton L., Laurillard D. Trends in research on student learning. *Studies in Higher Education* **4** (1): 87–101. 1979.
4. Fenwick T. Rethinking processes of adult learning. Draft material for a chapter in *Understanding Adult Education and Training*, 3rd edition. 2003. Available at: www.ualberta.ca/~tfenwick/ext/pubs/print/adultlearning.htm.
5. http://www.complexityandeducation.ualberta.ca/index.htm.
6. Cooper H., Braye S., Geyer R. Complexity and interprofessional education. *Learning in Health and Social Care* **3** (4): 179–189. 2004.
7. Apple M.W. *Official Knowledge: Democratic education in a conservative age.* New York: Routledge. 1993.
8. Osberg D.C., Biesta G.J.J., Cilliers P. From representation to emergence: complexity's challenge to the epistemology of schooling. *Educational Philos and Theory*, **39** (7) 2007/ In press.
9. Ulmer G. *Applied grammatology: post(e)-pedagogy from Jacques Derrida to Joseph Beuys.* Baltimore: Johns Hopkins University Press. 1985.
10. Biesta G.J.J. *Beyond Learning. Democratic education for a human future.* Boulder (CA): Paradigm Publishers. 2006.
11. Arendt H. *The Human Condition.* Chicago: University of Chicago Press. 1958.
12. Nancy JL. Introduction. In: *Who comes after the subject?* (ed J.L. Nancy), pp.1–8. New York: Routledge. 1991 p.7.

13. Biesta G.J.J. Radical intersubjectivity: reflections on the 'different' foundation of education. *Studies in Philosophy and Education* **18** (4): 203–220. 1999.

14. Thomas G. Theory's spell – on qualitative inquiry and educational research. *British Educational Research Journal* **28** (3): 419–435. 2002.

15. Law J., Urry J. Enacting the social. Department of Sociology and the Centre for Science Studies, Lancaster University, Lancaster. 2003. Available at: http://www.lancs.ac.uk/fss/sociology/research/resalph.htm#lr.

16. Ridley D. Puzzling experiences in higher education: critical moments for conversation. *Studies in Higher Education* **29** (1): 91–107. 2004.

17. Goodwin L. Resilient spirits; disadvantaged students making it at an elite university. London: Routledge Falmer. 2002.

18. Johnson S. *Emergence.* London: Penguin. 2001.

19. Byrne D. Focusing on the case in quantitative and qualitative research. ESRC Research Methods Programme, Workshop 4, The Case Study, 12–13 January 2005.

20. Goldstein J. Impetus without teleology: the self-transcending construction of emergence. Paper given at the Complexity, Science and Society Conference, Liverpool, September 2005.

21. Byrne D. Complexity, configurations and cases. *Theory, Culture and Society* **22** (5): 95–111. 2005.

22. Haggis T. Meaning, identity and 'motivation': expanding what matters in understanding learning in higher education? *Studies in Higher Education* **29** (3): 335–352. 2004.

23. Haggis T. Researching difference and particularity: new perspectives from complexity theory. Paper given at Challenging the Orthodoxies in Educational Research, Middlesex University, London, December 2005.

24. Donald M. *A Mind So Rare: The evolution of human consciousness.* New York and London: W.W. Norton. 2001.

25. Merleau-Ponty M. *Phenomenology of Perception*, C. Smith (trans.), with revisions by Williams F., Gurriére D. London: Routledge. 1989.

26. Edelman G. *Wider Than the Sky: The phenomenal gift of consciousness.* New Haven: Yale University Press. 2004.

27. Thompson E. Editor's introduction: empathy and consciousness. *Journal of Consciousness Studies* **8** (5–7): 1–32. 2001.

28. Johnson S. *Mind Wide Open: Your brain and the neuroscience of everyday life.* New York: Scribner. 2004.

29. Ramachadran V.S. *A Brief Tour of Human Consciousness: From imposter poodles to purple numbers.* New York: Pi Press. 2004.

30. Lodge D. *Consciousness and the Novel.* New York and London: Penguin Books. 2002.

31. Woolf V. *Mrs. Dalloway.* London: Chancellor Press. 1925 and 1994, p.179.

32. Cunningham M. *The Hours.* New York: Picador. 1998 pp.34–35.

33. Iftody T., Sumara D., Davis B. Consciousness and the literary engagement: toward a bio-cultural theory of reading and learning. *Language and Literacy* **8** (1). Available from http://www.langandlit.ualberta.ca/. 2006.

34. Luce-Kapler R., Dobson T., Sumara D. *et al.* E-literature and the digital engagement of consciousness. Article in press. 2006.

35. Davis B. *Inventions of Teaching: A genealogy.* Mahwh, New Jersey: Lawrence Erlbaum. 2004.

CHAPTER 5

Health and complexity

Edited by Rod Lambert, Ceri Brown and Jan Bogg

Introduction

Complexity science is being used in the domain of clinical healthcare organisation to understand how processes interact and produce change. This description of a complex adaptive system (CAS) differs significantly from an understanding of a system using a Newtonian view. Briefly, a Newtonian system possesses three features: reductionism, linearity and hierarchy. Reductionism implies that the whole system can be understood by an examination of all of its constituent parts, such as a clock mechanism [Arthur in [1]: p.334]. Linearity implies that cause and effect are known and that a known stimulus produces a repeatable effect. Hierarchy suggests the concept of control under the gaze of a 'director' of action within the system.

In a CAS, its elements undergo a continual 'kaleidoscopic array of simultaneous nonlinear interactions' [2], which gives rise to system properties different from the Newtonian. Firstly, the behaviour of the whole system cannot be understood by examination of its constituent parts because of multiple interactions between the parts. In complexity, the behaviour of the whole system is said to be 'emergent.' Nonlinearity is observed because repeated stimuli produce differing effects owing to the interrelationships between the elements changing over time. Complex systems are non-hierarchical because the observed pattern of behaviour develops from interactions between agents: systems self-organise.

Complexity in healthcare

An example from the recent past of the National Health Service (NHS) illustrates the dominance of Newtonian thinking. The Labour Government elected in 1997 made an election pledge to reduce the number of patients on surgical waiting lists. Despite government policy and financial investment, the waiting list statistics changed very slowly, and in May 1998 the Secretary of State for Health, Frank Dobson, stated:

> 'I said last year that the waiting lists were like a supertanker. It would take time to slow them down, longer to bring them to a stop, and even longer to turn them around' [3].

The explicit use of the metaphor 'supertanker' for 'NHS waiting lists' suggests many associations: a captain on the bridge giving orders which are obeyed by subordinates, reliable and unchanging linkages between the systems of the ship, and a slow but linear response to the turn of the helm. Action towards embracing a more systematic approach to providing a detailed analysis of multiple influences on health and the provision of healthcare has therefore been slow to become accepted and established. However, on 28 February 2006, an article appeared on the front page of *The Times* [4], showing a complex diagram from the National Audit Office [5] of the diverse influences on obesity in childhood (Figure 5.1). This provided a recent example of how multiple interactions are beginning to be considered, and may be informing healthcare decisions and clinical practice in the UK.

The first major attempt to promote ideas from complexity science into healthcare was in a series of four articles published in the *British Medical Journal* in 2001 [6–9]. The first of these [6] helped those unfamiliar with complexity to understand basic theoretical concepts and linked these to clinical examples. The second article examined the application of these initial concepts to clinical understanding and

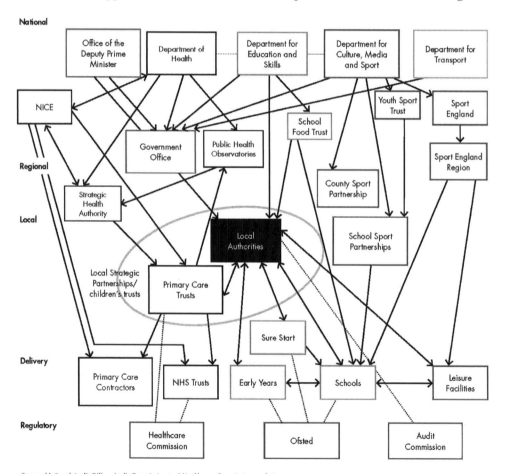

Source: National Audit Office, Audit Commission and Healthcare Commission analysis.

Figure 5.1. Tackling child obesity.

decision-making in situations such as glycaemic control, uncertainty in diagnosis and health promotion [7]. The third article [8] concentrated on how complex systems can function within management settings and the implications for leadership styles and roles. The final article [9] provided insights into how complexity science can be used to promote education and training of healthcare professionals through which to encourage a consideration of wider issues when making clinical judgements. At about the same time as these articles were published, there was evidence of increased interest in the concept of complexity in healthcare with the development in 2000 of a group calling themselves the 'Tufton Group' owing to the location in London of their meeting place, but with a more formal title of the 'Complexity in Primary Care Group'. The group still holds meetings, although the venue has recently changed to the University of Warwick. The group considers many clinical and management issues, particularly with a focus on primary care. An annual conference of the Exeter Health Complexity Group has been held since 2001, and books on complexity and its association to healthcare issues have been produced by members of these groups [10–12]. When in 2005 the University of Liverpool began to develop its 'Complexity Science and Society' conference, this provided a natural forum through which to further develop the links across members of the healthcare professions with an interest in complexity science.

This chapter provides an indication of the areas of interest, and the major developments taking place that continue to consider that complexity science can inform healthcare. The general areas remain similar to those indicated in the initial *British Medical Journal* articles, with sections in this chapter considering healthcare management and leadership, primary care and clinical applications. These demonstrate that not only is complexity science being developed in different ways within healthcare, but that its implications are potentially far reaching and provide exciting opportunities for a new look at the influences on health and healthcare.

Management and leadership complexity in healthcare

The NHS is a very large organisation, in which styles of management and leadership have changed as often as there have been policy changes. This section begins with an overview by Rihani of how the organisation is influenced by the presence of 'arms-length bodies' and how a complexity approach may be considered as an appropriate way forward. McMillan then considers the potential use of two different models to examine how complexity thinking may be operationalised in a management setting and how this can influence leadership styles. Merali then offers an insight into how CASs can be used to identify the nodes and connectivity within healthcare management, enhancing our ability to maximise management responsiveness in the present day, in a way that will maximise best practice in the future. In the final contribution to this section, Sturmberg and Martin present a 'vortex model' to examine how complexity can influence policy makers in recognising that personal health is experienced and alters differently with everyone.

NHS: anarchy or perfection?
Samir Rihani

The NHS is being torn apart by two contradictory visions. On the one hand, there is positivist thinking, launched by Descartes centuries ago, which remains the favoured option to this day. Command-and-control mediated through a steep hierarchical structure and enforced by an elaborate inspection and regulation bureaucracy is the model of choice here.

On the other hand, evidence nowadays suggests that healthcare and the way it is managed behave as CASs. Soft management methods are required in this instance based on considerable local autonomy, trial and error, shared learning, minimal central control, and active participation by all stakeholders.

The NHS is not unaware of complexity and its arcane ways. A brief glance at NHS publications reveals the major strides already taken towards a shift to complexity thinking. And here lies the problem: thinking and doing are out of step.

At base, this process of change presents an unbearable challenge not to frontline staff but to those at the top who stand to lose most of their power and influence. The shock waves go well beyond secretaries of state, ministers, chief executives and senior civil servants to engulf a vast superstructure of organisations that have come into being, mostly for good reasons, over many decades.

The so-called 'arms-length bodies' (ALBs) give an idea of the extent of the upheaval. Plans were adopted in 2004 to reduce their number down to 20 (from 40) by 2007/08. However, those remaining present a formidable central force that employs over 18,000 people and costs more than £4 billion annually. They will continue to flood frontline organisations with demands for actions and extensive form filling that generates time-consuming site visits, which in turn results in more information collection and work.

The ALBs are not the only source of extraneous work that encroaches on the ability of frontline organisations to undertake their fundamental task of looking after the needs of their community. There are about 100 professional committees that also act as generators of work.

Why do they create an endless stream of work? Basically, they have to present new ideas all the while to the Department of Health and the NHS to remain in business. Otherwise, what is the point of having an ALB? Does this mean all ALBs are unnecessary or counterproductive? Not at all: some are indispensable, but others are the product of an outdated mechanistic vision of healthcare.

Adoption of a complexity framework in healthcare is not going to be easy. Apart from the natural tendency for governments to seek to retain their hold on power, radical transformation will threaten numerous organisations and links that have been forged over many decades. The ongoing effort to reduce ALBs down to 20, originally started in 1997 when New Labour came to power, gives an indication of the scale of task that would have to be tackled. Nonetheless, with ever-increasing complexity and the attendant failure of current practices, the project is unavoidable.

Riding the waves of change: using complex adaptive processes
Elizabeth McMillan

Issues related to change and uncertainty are high on all organisational agendas and present challenging situations for all healthcare managers. Complexity science recognises that we do not live in a stable predictable world and it offers fresh thinking for managers seeking to work successfully with fast flowing uncertainties. This section focuses on two useful models: dancing on 'the edge of chaos' and the complex adaptive process model.

Dancing on the Edge of Chaos

As Figure 5.2 shows, living species, including CASs, are able to exist in a spectrum of situations ranging from the orderly and highly stable to the disorderly or chaotic. Research has shown that systems are most successful, innovative and flexible when they operate close to the chaotic area, or 'on the edge of chaos'. Many large bureaucracies live too close to the stable zone and are at risk of ossification. Other organisations, such as the early dotcoms, live in the chaos zone and risk disintegration. Thus successful organisations need to learn to 'dance' on the edge of chaos. Sometimes they may need to dip into the stable zone if things are getting too disorderly or they may need to introduce novelty and innovation if there is risk of ossification.

The danger is if an organisation or an individual becomes stuck in either of the extremes. Managers may use this model as an analytical tool to consider the overall situation in which they find themselves and to either increase or reduce novelty.

CASs have evolved over the millennia in a survival response to a world that is constantly changing in unpredictable and often hostile ways. They offer organisations and managers a blueprint for survival that is based on inherent human behaviours. Figure 5.3, the complex adaptive process model, is based on research and consultancy, and it provides managers with a conceptual and an analytical tool that will enable them to behave as CASs and thus fulfil their potential to operate

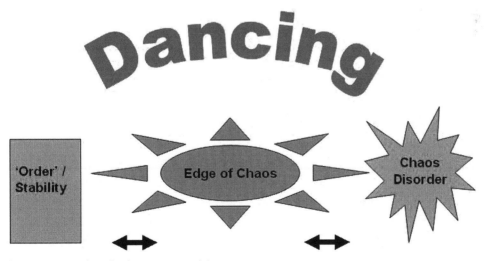

Figure 5.2. Complex adaptive process model.

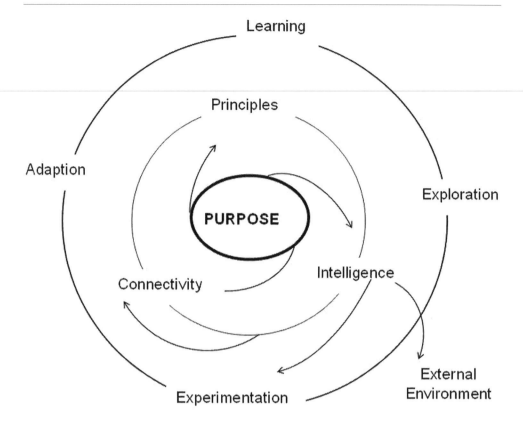

Figure 5.3. Complex adaptive process model.

successfully in a complex and uncertain world. CASs are always *exploring* their environments, seeking information and *intelligence* to inform their actions. They *experiment* with new ideas and actions, *adapt* and *learn* as they interact with each other and their environments. All individuals in the system are closely *connected* and interact in a nonlinear way. There is no centralised control, but a strongly shared *purpose* drives their actions and they are guided by underlying and shared *principles*.

Managers may compare their own processes with those of the model. It may also be used to suggest new possibilities for change by placing the appropriate purpose in the central circle and then enacting the different stages of the process. It may also be used in much the same way to set up projects, help deliver them and later appraise them.

'Jam today': complexity theory and managing in the present
Yasmin Merali

The NHS is increasingly recognising the importance of networking. However, because of an excessive focus on efficient process delivery, it undermines the organisation's adaptive potential. An increasingly popular metaphor for the NHS is that of the CAS, inherently stable and able to adapt to changes in its operating context as it meets them. A CAS is characterised by emergence and self-organisation. The efficient operation of such a system is predicated on the network form of organising.

Fundamentally, a network is a collection of nodes interconnected by a set of links. In practice, at any given time, nodes are selectively connected to other nodes in the network: a snapshot of the network form of CAS organisation looks like a network of networks – constellations of tightly connected nodes linked with other (distant and proximate) nodes. The response flexibility of the CAS arises from its ability to change the connectivity (links) and membership (nodes) within and between individual network constellations.

The network form of organising allows the CAS to use 'real-time intelligence' (information about local contingencies as they arise) to respond to environmental threats and opportunities as it meets them by selectively configuring and mobilising particular constellations of networks and resources [13]. The defining feature of these networks is that the 'design' enables dynamic networking. The inherent potential networking capability confers both agility and efficiency of resource deployment to respond to contingencies. Boundary nodes (those exposed to, and interacting with, the external environment) signal perturbations in the environment. The interdependence of network nodes and clusters for survival (the survival of the functioning individual both maintains and is maintained by the persistence of the CAS as a whole) results in mutual accommodation of nodes, and presents the phenomenon of collective, distributed regulation and control of internal co-ordination and consistency.

Networks figure strongly in NHS management rhetoric. Attempts are being made to design services for seamless inter-organisational delivery. However, the focus is on efficient process delivery, and the approach is one of engineering 'hard-wired' networks: the most efficient paths for current 'best practice' processes are implemented. Standards and protocols are set at the most detailed level to ensure conformance. These networks are in danger of becoming 'over-engineered' sclerotic structures. The intent to achieve a universal, demonstrable (by conformance to standard targets) best-practice NHS equates to the White Queen's[1] logic of 'jam tomorrow' and produces the Red Queen effect[2]. Best practice extrapolated from yesterday's experience is tomorrow's 'past practice'. The diversion of resources to achieve the established best practice ideal by some 'target date' channels current efforts so strongly that there is no opportunity to harness resources for 'good enough' practice to address today's local needs, while keeping open the potential for adaptation to tomorrow's contingencies.

When the future is uncertain, goal-orientated strategies of managing on the trajectory from the past state to some desired future state (with the present merely plotted as some point on the pre-defined graph) is limiting. How we manage the present circumscribes the potentiality open to us in the future.

CAS networks are the connectors and repositories of current capabilities and mechanisms for the gestation and dynamic realisation of the requisite variety of

---

1 This refers to the White Queen's proclamation in Lewis Caroll's *Through the Looking Glass* [14]. When Alice declines to have her wages paid in jam, the White Queen becomes irate and says, 'You could not have it today anyway, because we have jam every other day. We had jam yesterday and we have jam tomorrow, but never jam today'.
2 This refers to the Red Queen's quote in *Through the Looking Glass*: 'Now, here, you see, it takes all the running you can do to keep in the same place'.

responses for contingencies as we meet them. Exploiting the potential for dynamism afforded by the network form of organising in the NHS entails going beyond process design to address organisational design. This requires a shift from paradigms predicated on managerially designed alignment of structure and function, to ones predicated on designing the requisite networking potential for dynamic alignment of capabilities and resources with contingencies for coordinated action.

The healthcare vortex: understanding health, healthcare and healthcare policy as a complex adaptive system
Joachim P. Sturmberg and Carmel M. Martin

Health at the centre of healthcare

Personal health can be understood as an individual's adaptive experience within the framework of a CAS [15]. Patterns of individual health are central to the work of healthcare systems, as they determine community and population health outcomes. To fully appreciate the complexities of the personal health experience, it is necessary to appreciate the levelled experiences of human beings [16]. Personal experiences of health emerge from sense-making about body and mind sensations, and the social and psychological framing of those sensations into illness or health.

A well-functioning health system must focus on optimising personal health, i.e. the improvement or maintenance of the personal health status [17], rather than merely the reduction or elimination of a particular disease. This interconnected nature of personal health is known as the somato-psycho-socio-semiotic model of health [15].

The goal of achieving the greatest possible health gain means that health service planners must allow individual health services to self-organise, based on local and individual needs, by fostering strong relationships and learning attitudes among all healthcare providers [18].

The healthcare vortex – a metaphor to understand healthcare in context

A vortex is a useful metaphor to describe CASs. A vortex demonstrates the interconnectedness of pattern, structure and process. Structure and process co-exist and co-evolve, and despite constant change the property of self-stabilisation maintains the vortex close to its original state[3] [19]. In organisational language, this property is reflected in the core value of the organisation: in this case personal health.

Using the vortex metaphor we suggest that principally healthcare must be structured, as illustrated in Figure 5.4. All activities within the vortex ultimately determine the personal health status, represented at the bottom of the vortex.

The different levels within the vortex describe various functional dimensions of the healthcare system. The top describes the socio-political level where policy decision making resides. The policy framework at that level moves to the local area health level at which health professionals and local health bureaucrats determine how to translate the policies into local delivery models and thus will vary according to local circumstances. Local healthcare providers, in their individual consultations, will finally deliver services reflecting the overall policy. Here again the way of delivery

---

3 We all have been fascinated by this phenomenon, playing with the vortex in the bathtub.

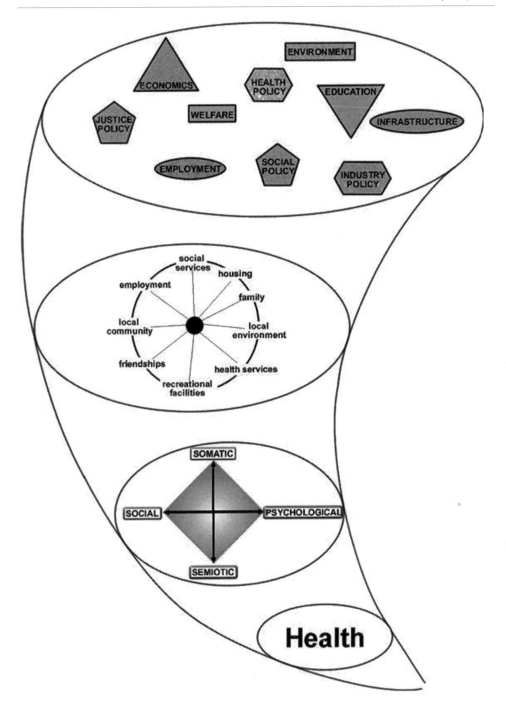

Figure 5.4. The healthcare vortex.

will be unique for each provider and unique to each individual, leading to the best possible – and most appropriate – health gain for each patient. Nonlinearity allows 'different' but mutually agreeable outcomes to emerge, and feedback helps to modulate the activities at all levels: further properties of CASs[4].

Utilising the healthcare vortex in health service planning

The vortex metaphor helps health service planning to re-focus on health. It forces us to acknowledge that health is experienced differently by individuals and that the experience may change over time. Equally it forces health service planners to acknowledge that successful health policy is significantly influenced by policy decisions in other portfolios.

Most importantly, however, loss of personal health – and particularly loss of health of whole communities – reflects a disturbance of the system at all its levels.

Complexity in primary care

Having identified some of the management issues within the vast organisation of healthcare, an important subset of this organisation is primary care. A commonly accepted definition of primary care is 'that level of a health service that provides entry into the system for all new needs and problems, provides person-focused (not disease oriented) care over time, provides care for all but very uncommon or unusual conditions, and coordinates or integrates care provided elsewhere or by others' [20: pp.8–9]. This section begins with Innes' examination of complexities existing in the consultation between doctor and patient. Martin and Sturmberg consider the broad nature of primary healthcare reforms and their limitations, identifying the need for more realistic and complex modelling of primary care systems for effective planning and policy reform. These two perspectives provide a clear view of how linear thinking restricts progress in primary healthcare provision, and how the use of a complexity model may free practitioners to more actively engage with the complexities of everyday clinical practice.

The consultation as a complex adaptive system
Andrew Innes

The consultation between doctors and patients is the cornerstone of clinical practice. Through this process problems are defined and solutions sought. This has traditionally been seen in a positivist context, but can the consultation be considered as a complex system? And, if such a concept is tenable, then what might it mean for our understanding of the consultation and what are the implications of such a view?

A recent paper has advanced a theoretical critique of the consultation as a CAS [21]. Through the lens of complexity theory, consultations are seen as complex processes where meaning emerges often unpredictably from the interaction between the clinician and the patient. The role of the clinician therefore becomes that of an enquiring participant who seeks to influence change in a patient's condition. More recently, a focus group study has been undertaken by the same authors to examine

---

4 There are many roads leading to Rome.

whether general practitioners and patients talk about consultations in a way that is consistent with understanding them as complex systems [22]. In this study, patients and doctors were invited to talk about various aspects of consultations, and the transcripts were analysed by using a complexity framework.

From a theoretical perspective, diversity of agents is the key to understanding CASs. Many influences can be seen to have agency in consultations either by virtue of their presence in the consultation, for example computers in the consulting room, or through the individuals present as for example in the prior 'organising experiences' of patients and doctors[5]. Complexity theory offers an account of agency in its own right but also one that is able to incorporate the meaning of agency implied within social science, i.e. the idea that the agency of individuals is limited by social structures. The difference is that the interaction between agents, and between agents and structures, is dynamically nonlinear and produces outcomes that are unpredictable and sensitive to the unique circumstances of individual consultations.

Nonlinearity is an important feature of complex systems making them inherently unpredictable and is a recognisable characteristic of some consultations. Numerous small influences in consultations can have large effects and vice versa. For patients, nonlinearity seems to be equated with individuality of their particular circumstances. Attractors can also be identified within consultations; for example, the influence of a computer template for a chronic disease on the treatment a patient receives and the clinical approach adopted by the doctor. Diagnosis and diagnostic labelling can also impose attractors on patients' experiences.

Complexity theory describes a state known as the 'edge of chaos,' where a complex system is unstable and sensitive to change. Some consultations have this form of instability. Indeed, a doctor or patient may move a consultation to the 'edge of chaos' as a deliberate strategy to achieve greater creativity. Actions by doctors or patients or the intrinsic nature of clinical problems such as substance misuse can cause consultations to move towards this zone. The risks of consulting in this zone are high and often to the doctor–patient relationship, but the rewards in terms of effecting useful change are considerable.

General practitioners recognise that consultations are complex, both in the colloquial and, when informed, the theoretical sense: yet within a very constrained time-frame they have to discover solutions to health and social problems with their patients. The different contexts within which consultations take place also need to be considered. To assess and manage problems, general practitioners undertake a process of 'complexity filtering' and pattern recognition supported by use of clinical rules. This process of complexity filtering is most evident in consultations in emergency settings, where safety is the priority and the consultation is 'stripped down' to its basic clinical components.

Complexity theory does seem to offer a useful framework for the analysis of consultations, and both doctors and patients do discuss their experience of consultations in ways that are in tune with complexity thinking. Such an analysis is of practical use to doctors and those who teach doctors to consult. In particular, the

---

5   The term 'organising experience', first described by Ralph Stacey, denotes a previous experience that acts to determine current behaviour: for example, a patient with a sore throat who has previously attended his doctor and been prescribed antibiotics is likely to attend when he next experiences the same symptoms with the expectation that antibiotics will be prescribed once again.

'edge of chaos' is a risky but potentially creative zone in which consultations can take place.

Primary healthcare reform: a complexity perspective
Carmel Martin and Joachim Sturmberg

> *'Primary health care will continue to evolve, since many countries view it as a policy cornerstone'* [23].

Governments in the industrialised world are looking for solutions to improve their healthcare systems. Pressures to achieve better expenditure control and/or greater productivity and efficiency need to be balanced against deeply rooted moral imperatives to maintain universal access to necessary care, and to improve the equity with which services are distributed across social classes. Each government is challenged to make the system more responsive to user needs, and to bring the health system component parts and providers under particular financial control. Reforms are being contemplated, organised or implemented, sometimes in direct contradiction to other policy directions [23].

Starfield and others have repeatedly demonstrated that an emphasis of primary care – a generalist first contact level of service in a health system – is cost-effective compared with a secondary and tertiary care emphasis on observational studies. Primary healthcare, which incorporates primary care but takes a broad and intersectoral systems approach to addressing health determinants, is associated with lower costs and better outcomes internationally [24]. Thus, internationally, policy makers in recent years have embraced the importance of primary (health) care (PHC) as a key strategy [25].

Yet, there is often much disappointment from policy makers, providers, the public and lobby groups about the outcomes of PHC reforms and system performance. Internationally, reforms of PHC systems are continual, as reforms bring both improvements such as better management of some common diseases [26], and unintended consequences including little impact on widening health disparities [27], undesired shifts in care [28], low professional morale [29] and less public satisfaction with general practice [30].

Are there basic flaws in the conceptual understandings and knowledge of primary care and health-systems decisions about the nature of progress to better healthcare and health? Currently, a wide range of piecemeal assumptions, evidence and knowledge drive PHC change, which often lacks coherence.

We propose that PHC is a multi-levelled complex system connecting many types of activity and service, which is dynamic and constantly adapting around the concepts and demands for health and healthcare in a socio-political environment.

Complexity theories, studies and modelling are directed to understanding patterns which are not predictable by traditional evidence and social knowledge. Health systems are social systems and reforms are perturbations of these system that are typically fragmented and micro-level in concept without a detailed analysis of the patterns, structure and process in the whole. Misaligning types of knowledge and approaches with the nature of systems is likely to lead to ongoing and ineffective reforms and disjointed change without understanding the whole.

Reforms are inevitable as an adaptive process to changing environments, but unless they are set up as complex system change, they have the potential to shift care towards static or chaotic patterns. Appropriate complex social systems models, pattern analysis and modelling in planning, monitoring and refining reforms with the stakeholder are required.

Complex systems provide a framework for an expanded knowledge base, debate and discussion of reforms and development of PHC goals and strategies [31].

Clinical applications of complexity in healthcare

Any consideration of theoretical constructs in healthcare would be incomplete if it did not consider clinical implications. Brown begins this section with a consideration of chronic pain, concluding that when applying a complex systems approach, it is necessary to identify rules and patterns that influence the system before trying to effect change. Lambert considers the application of a complexity model to panic disorder, enabling system components to be identified, and for different points of entry into the system to be identified through which treatment may be effective. Rabone *et al.* demonstrate how an everyday procedure like disinfection, when viewed in detail, also demonstrates complex patterns. Watson identifies the complex range of influences on gait retraining after traumatic brain injury, Deakin *et al.* show how using chromatic information can help to monitor systems (including human systems), and Holt considers complex interactions influencing blood glucose levels in diabetic patients.

Chronic pain through the lens of complexity
Cary Brown

It is increasingly emphasised that people are complex biological systems that do not behave in a linear fashion [32–34], and that effective healthcare for the growing number of chronic disease and lifestyle issues must be grounded in a non-reductionist paradigm focused on understanding relationships and taking a flexible approach to problem-solving [35–38]. Of particular concern is the experience of chronic pain, the prevalence of which has been cited as between 12–35% of the population at any one time, and between 49% and 80% across the lifespan [39]. The authors concluded that chronic back pain alone is one of the most costly conditions for which the economics have been analysed in the UK, yet it accounts for potentially as little as 16% of benign pain conditions, representing only the tip of the iceberg in the total economic costs of chronic pain [40]. Finding a consistently accepted definition of chronic pain is problematic and has been cited as one of the features contributing to the ongoing problems in effective intervention for people with persistent pain [41]. Depending on the theoretical perspective, definitions range from malfunctioning auto-immune systems, to conversion reactions triggered by abuse, to an adaptive response to threatened livelihood and loss of income. However, two consistent features across theoretical perspectives are temporality and unexpectedness; in other words, pain that is unexpected and lasts longer than expected.

In a study investigating the lack of congruence between service users' and service providers' beliefs about which treatments are important for chronic pain, Brown [42:

p.42] used a policy delphi method to determine if study participants endorsed reframing chronic pain within a CAS's perspective [37]. Their responses revealed conflicting beliefs that, although chronic pain had several elements consistent with a CAS, also demonstrated several strong linear elements. Additionally, participants saw chronic pain as lacking both predictability and certainty.

When CAS theory was applied to the findings, paradoxical beliefs emerged. Complexity theory proposes that paradox in itself is not the problem. Rather, the problem lies in how an organisation deals with this inherent feature of the system. From a linear perspective, efforts generally target reducing the occurrence of perceived problems (like paradoxical beliefs) and harmonisation of opinion. Ironically, paradoxical beliefs actually increase as ineffective linear efforts are applied to complex problems in futile efforts to encourage homogeneity of beliefs and practices [43: p.11]. When linear problem-solving focuses on resolving this type of paradox, it generates a cumulative feedback loop where increased input (resources expended in an effort to reduce paradoxical beliefs) actually results in increased output (chronicity of the pain experience in the case of Brown's study) [41].

CAS theory proposes that organisations must foster the perspective that paradoxes, for example: *'everyone deserves treatment/we cannot afford to treat everyone'* and *'opiates help relieve pain symptoms/opiates lead to addiction'*, can never be resolved but they can be lived with. Zimmerman [45] states that to facilitate adaptive and positive change in complex systems we should expect and use the unexpected. This attitude towards conflict does not come easily and poor skills in understanding and using conflict creatively will interfere with the ability to take on new policies and behaviours [46].

Gordon and Dahl [47] speculate that in chronic pain management there is an overall failure to see change proportionate to the effort exerted because the wrong questions are being asked. They state that people do not necessarily need more information about the methods and technical aspects of pain management, but rather about interactions within the system itself. They suggest that continuing to examine what are actually systems' problems with clinical tools is akin to trying to break the sound barrier by tinkering with a Model-T Ford car. Plsek *et al.* [45] propose that developing simple rules and minimum specifications (as opposed to exhaustive criteria and regulations) are key to successful management of change in complex systems. In the case of chronic pain, we need to first identify the existing patterns and rules that promote chronicity before seeking to effect change within the system.

By applying the principles of complexity theory to identify as yet often hidden patterns and simple rules, stakeholders can be guided to dealing overtly, transparently and constructively with disagreement and paradox. This, in turn, can generate positive and creative change across the chronic pain experience.

Complexity, panic and primary care
Rod Lambert

About 90% of mental healthcare is provided in primary care. However, only 30–50% of these problems are currently recognised, and outcomes from treatment are sometimes poor. A large unrecognised population of people with mental health problems therefore continues to be vulnerable, take time off work, and experience social, psychological and physical consequences [48]. In England, the cost of mental illness in 2002/3 was estimated at over £77 billion per year, including the costs of care provided by the NHS, local authorities, privately funded services, family and friends; lost output in the economy caused by people being unable to work (paid and unpaid) and the human costs of reduced quality of life, and loss of life, amongst those experiencing a mental health problem [49]. The most common treatments for mental health problems are either medication or psychological therapies (alone or in combination). The National Service Framework for Mental Health identifies, however, that there is an inter-relationship between mental health and lifestyle factors. These factors include smoking, excess alcohol consumption, drug use, exercise and general physical health, and suggest that these provide possible mechanisms through which both health promotion and treatment can be approached.

Panic disorder (PD) is a severe form of anxiety affecting about 1.5% of the population, with this being relatively consistent across cultures [50] and is seen regularly within primary care settings. It represents an often chronic problem with high healthcare resource use, particularly in terms of GP time, medication costs and referral for clinical investigations. However, possible causes of PD may include environmental, cognitive and personality factors; genetic inheritance and neurobiological factors such as the influence of neurotransmitters, body systems and lifestyle-related factors. These factors interact in ways that meet [51] a definition of a CAS. Viewing the development of mental health problems, such as PD, in more dynamic multifactorial terms promotes clinical reasoning which considers the influences of the additive effect of multiple factors.

By identifying the diverse agents influencing the development of mental health problems, it becomes possible to examine potential therapeutic mechanisms through which to identify and influence system-tipping points. Applying this approach to PD promotes a deeper understanding of the underlying processes, and the condition itself can begin to be viewed from a different perspective.

For example, Figure 5.5 shows that a panic reaction can be viewed as a pattern of behaviour (attractor) that may be reinforced by repeated experience (forming deeper

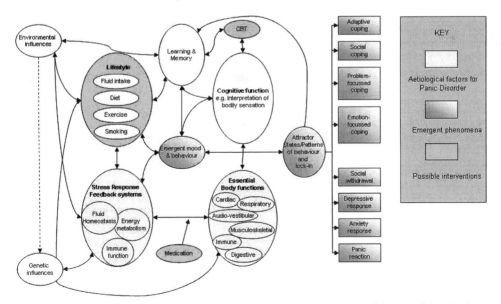

Figure 5.5. Complex interactions and panic disorder: emergent phenomena and therapeutic implications.

attractor wells), which can be influenced by a range of internal and external factors. Therefore, by viewing the system within which panic disorder develops as complex, it can offer an explanation of how and why a range of traditional treatment interventions (including medication and CBT) can be effective, and also how interventions such as lifestyle review can influence patient outcomes and increase patient control over symptoms by influencing different parts of the system.

Is this merely conjecture? A recent randomised controlled trial [52] compared a lifestyle approach with routine general practitioner care of the treatment of PD in primary care. The results showed that after 16 weeks of treatment, patients in the lifestyle arm showed a reduction from a mean Beck Anxiety Inventory (BAI) score of 29.5 (severe anxiety) to a mean of 9.2 (mild anxiety), compared with 29.4 to 17.2 (moderate anxiety) in the GP care arm ($p=0.004$, 95% confidence interval mean difference = -9.8, -15.1 to -4.6). Scores at a 10-month follow-up were not statistically significant, however, and this approach requires further investigation. Effect sizes were very similar to those obtained from cognitive behavioural therapy, and showed improved results compared with some studies of medication. Although not conclusive, these results indicate that applying a complexity-based aetiological model to mental health problems can identify broader influences on patient experiences and also suggest possible points of input to the system that can effect positive symptom control and change.

Is disinfection chaotic?
Kenneth L. Rabone, Jonathan K. Rabone and Jeremy A.L. Rabone

Disinfection to control pathogenic microbes (i.e. those that cause disease) is important in society and there is currently a concern that such control may be inadequate in hospitals to prevent nosocomial infections (i.e. infections acquired in hospital).

Denyer and Stewart [53] have reviewed the mechanisms by which disinfectants act. They regard most disinfectants as chemical biocides with a relative lack of selectivity. The vegetative bacterial cell presents three broad regions for biocide interaction: the cell wall, the cytoplasmic membrane and the cytoplasm. The target most frequently cited in the biocide literature is the cytoplasmic membrane.

Disinfection has a specific meaning: a reduction in microbial numbers from about 10^8 cells per millilitre to 10^3 cells per millilitre or fewer at 20°C for five microbial types in a standard test (European Suspension Test [54]). The parameter calculated is the decadic logarithm of the ratio of microbial numbers before and after the procedure, and disinfection is achieved therefore when a value of at least 5 is obtained. The precision of this test is extremely low [55, 56] and so far no-one has given a convincing explanation as to why this should be so.

Computer simulations using a cellular automata approach [57] suggest that the variability in microbial disinfection may depend on initial conditions and the dynamics of mixing. Microbial cell death can result from the catastrophic collapse of the cytoplasmic membrane of the cell as the biocide is concentrated in that membrane by physico-chemical partition and reaches some critical concentration. To get to the membrane, the biocide must first adsorb at the cell wall and then diffuse through it [58].

Disinfection is therefore a complex process with a catastrophic event which is likely to be a phase change in the membrane caused by the disinfecting agent. This suggests that disinfection may be a chaotic process [59] and the test variability observed merely a reflection of its pseudo-random nature.

The reliability of microbiocide activity measurement can be improved by using a categorical or binary approach in combination with logistic regression to return an explicit probability for disinfection [60]. An advantage of the approach is that it lends itself to a cost-effective microplate format that simplifies testing and increases throughput with automated data capture and processing.

The authors acknowledge the contributions of Dr Mojgan Naeeni, Mr Michael Hoptroff and Mr Andrew Mitchell, all of Unilever Research and Development, Port Sunlight, Wirral, UK.

Complexity in therapist–patient interactions: an exploratory model using neurological physiotherapy and movement disorders as an example
Martin Watson

Many neurological physiotherapists work primarily to retrain movement in people with acquired brain injury. There is a growing body of evidence for the clinical effectiveness of their interventions [61]. What is sometimes less clear is which component(s) of the patient/therapist interaction lead to treatment success.

Current research projects which the writer and colleagues are involved with are investigating the effects of lycra orthoses on movement control problems experienced by brain-injured adults. These elasticated garments are prescribed as an adjunct to movement retraining when uncoordination and muscle weakness are problems [62]. One offshoot of this work has been to emphasise the complexity of the successful patient/therapist interaction. For example, upper limb orthoses, applied to help with reach/grasp difficulties, sometimes appear to help a subject's gait.

There are obvious reasons why treatment aimed at the upper limb might affect behaviour in the lower limb; e.g. the complex interconnecting biomechanical linkages between different segments of the moving body. However, further consideration of the issue led to the generation of a 'bigger picture' wherein an attempt was made to identify all possible influencing factors. Unsurprisingly, this 'influence diagram' (Figure 5.6) contains many features typical of a CAS, including recurrency and iterative positive feedback loops, lower level interactions, sensitivity to initial conditions, and the possibility that small changes in one part of the system may (sometimes) have more significant effects elsewhere. Components of this model include:

- entry into a clinical trial means that the patient is regularly exposed once more to a therapy/treatment environment;
- (renewed) interventions and/or exposure (re)focuses the subject on the nature of his/her motor impairments, reversing the effects of learned disuse;
- the patient perceives success, improvement and change, which in turn begets more success and improvement;
- success in the patient facilitates positivity in the therapist, which in turn enhances the enthusiasm with which treatment is delivered;
- success in the patient leads to positive feelings in relatives/carers, who in turn encourage the patient.

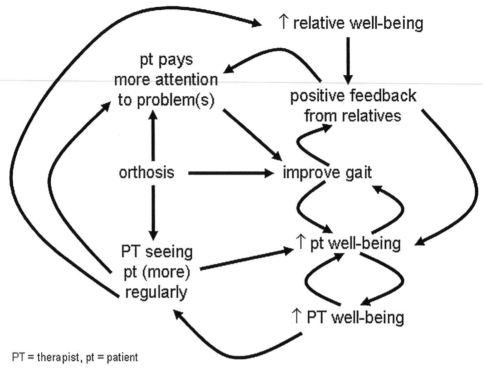

PT = therapist, pt = patient

Figure 5.6. Complexity model for gait change.

Most of the components of the model are obvious. However, like all CASs, it is the potential and multiple interactions of these (and probably other) components that may lead to the resulting emergent behaviour: a successful treatment outcome. Some of the components may be overtly manipulated by the clinician, whereas others may remain 'hidden'. All interactions will have a potential weighting, which can vary between occasions, individuals and circumstances. Subjects may thus sometimes show unexpected results; some may make sudden changes due to relatively minor (though innovative) interventions [63], whereas others may escape from the long-term stasis of a deep attractor well when there are (later) changes in circumstances [64].

As a final thought, the model may be said to do no more than identify many of the individual components of the placebo effect. This effect is, however, a powerful contributor to many if not all interventions that health professionals deliver [65]. Complexity theory may provide an ideal way to conceptualise the real world dynamics of the patient–therapist interaction.

Polychromatic modelling of complex biological factors: clinical applications
Anthony G. Deakin, Joseph W. Spencer and Gordon R. Jones

Engineering realises functionality through design within constraints such as aesthetics, ergonomics, time, cost and materials. For example, bridge-building is a complicated design process involving specification of components, interconnections, lifespan and maintenance, a process common across many areas such as construction, electrical engineering, electronics and software development. Each of these areas requires goal definition and solution implementation.

Bridges or electronic circuits are, however, parts in increasingly complex systems whose many components may interact unpredictably, as with the unanticipated oscillations of the Millennium Bridge: 'Individual patterns of response vary but the majority of the crowd interacts with the surface and with each other to develop substantial synchronised lateral movement' [66]. Similarly, electricity grids can produce emergent behaviour: 'sudden catastrophic blackouts caused by the effects of minor component failures rippling through an electricity network' [67]; complex systems functioning at the edge of chaos [68]. Natural systems have self-regulation known as homeostasis [69]; man-made systems, e.g. the Internet, also have regulation. The shared goal of natural and man-made systems alike is ensuring that their behaviour conforms to expectations, predicting *when* to intervene with routine examination, screening, planned maintenance or condition monitoring to assure system health.

The Centre for Intelligent Monitoring Systems' (CIMS) innovative *chromatic* approach, known as chromaticity [70], relates to the way the human vision system acquires/abstracts information: colour, brightness, contrast, shape, movement in objects. It has applications such as monitoring neonatal skin colour indicating levels of bilirubin, blood oxygenation and anaemia; temperature from colour changes in thermochromic material [71]; and colour yielding pH in biological systems [72]. Chromaticity extends to the acoustic domain, sound being processed for its characteristic dominant frequency, bandwidth and energy, just as dominant colour (hue), purity (saturation) and brightness (lightness) are obtained from visible phenomena. Indeed, chromaticity applies to *any* signal/spectrum from *any* domain to yield chromatic information about frequency, time, space, colour and other, derived parameters in the information world relating to the physical world. In this way, information processing by human senses is extended to ultrasonic, infrared and radio-frequency domains. Chromaticity is generic, typically non-invasive, retrofittable and portable, applies to signals and data from existing instruments, e.g. electrocardiograph waveforms, or is incorporated directly into front-end sensors. It is used qualitatively and quantitatively and relates to statistics and fuzzy sets. Compared with black-box techniques (e.g. neural nets), it is readily traceable. Information from various domains is integrated into a picture of system behaviour based on cross-correlations of information sources, useful for addressing emergent behaviour in complex systems. Whereas reductionism looks at individual elements in a system, and thereby may miss emergent unanticipated behaviour at higher levels, the chromatic information picture builds from lower levels or domains to a top-level indicator of system health, e.g. red/amber/green status indication with prognosis and trend information.

Chromaticity usefully addresses complex system behaviour by abstracting and managing system information in an integrated manner, and acts as a bridge from reductionism to complexity. Applications include assessing vehicle driver tiredness from driving behaviour and the health of elderly residents from their activity patterns [73]. CSS 2005 [74] includes theoretical developments and applications of chromaticity: identification of complex movement patterns [75], signal processing in optical coherence tomography [76], monitoring complex biological factors [77], event probability description [78] and information extraction from complex data sets [79].

Nonlinear dynamics and blood glucose control
Tim Holt

The application of nonlinear time series analysis to physiological signals, a field particularly well studied in cardiology and in brain dynamics, has produced new insights into the meaning of 'complexity' in both health and disease. The typical conclusion is that disease and ageing lead to a loss of complexity, defined by apparently disorderly but in fact structured variability exhibiting high entropy but long-range correlations [80]. Perhaps surprisingly, this field of study has yet to make significant inroads into diabetes research, despite the fact that the control of blood glucose is all about 'sensitivity to initial conditions', predictability, and the balance between convergent and divergent dynamics.

Diabetes is characterised by a loss of both insulin production and of the regulation mechanism that maintains physiological glucose variation. A range of clinical syndromes are recognised. In type 1 diabetes, which inevitably leads to insulin dependence, the physiological control mechanisms (which require little conscious effort on the individual's part) are effectively lost. Replacing these mechanisms requires adaptive decision-making strategies – a major challenge for the individual – and usually depends on frequent self-monitoring of blood glucose levels. Tight control may increase quality of life and certainly reduces long-term complications, so patients have a strong incentive to learn how to respond to the results of self-monitoring in a productive way. However, the target mean blood glucose level is close to the 'hypoglycaemic' range in which dangerously low levels may occur. 'Sailing close to the wind' becomes an everyday fact of life for the motivated patient. Traditional linear models of control assume a baseline equilibrium state: minimising variation is then the goal of therapy, and the focus is on accuracy of measurement of blood glucose determinants. In contrast, a nonlinear model would recognise that *interactions* between blood glucose determinants produce an additional and irreducible source of unpredictability. Variation is then a natural, inherent property of the system, and adaptive feedback between physiological parameters and behaviour becomes the key to stability [81]. Although this variation may need to be minimised, understanding its structure achieves a new relevance.

The recent availability of blood glucose profiles using continuous subcutaneous monitors provides a means through which 'healthy' dynamics might be more adequately studied using indices from nonlinear time series analysis.

Whilst the range of possible factors determining blood glucose variation is wide, a relatively low-dimensional model involving a few core determinants might account for much of the behaviour. These determinants (which include insulin levels, dietary carbohydrate influx, exercise levels and insulin sensitivity) might be plotted in a 'phase space', along with the blood glucose level itself. Although most of these variables are not easily measurable accurately in real-life situations, the model provides for the analysis of blood glucose profiles using data embedding techniques that are well established in other fields [82: pp.308–311]. This may allow the reconstruction of the underlying attractor that is unique to the individual patient.

The concept of an 'attractor' as a unique description of the individual patient's profile leads to several potentially important insights: which patients are likely to benefit from frequent self-monitoring, and which should resist 'tampering' with the system (an important current funding issue for the NHS)? What are the time horizons over which blood glucose levels are predictable, and how do these relate to the frequency of self-monitoring appropriate to the individual? Can we redefine and more adequately quantify the traditional concept of 'brittleness' in a new way, based both on current monitoring technology and the developing methodology of nonlinear time-series analysis?

These issues have been explored through two Maths Masters projects as part of a developing collaborative research programme at the University of Warwick between the Medical School and the Institute of Mathematics. This collaboration led on directly from the University of Liverpool Complexity, Science and Society conference of 2005.

Conclusion

The diversity of approaches that have considered the use of complexity models as providing added perspectives on real-life management and clinical situations within healthcare suggests that these only represent the tip of the iceberg. Healthcare thinking is moving away from a reductionist model, and into a future that focuses on analysing the interplay of processes and outcomes. Complexity science appears to offer a paradigm within which to do so.

References

1. Lewin R. *Complexity: Life at the edge of chaos*. London: Phoenix. 1993.
2. Holland J.H. *Adaptation in natural and artificial systems: an introductory analysis with applications to biology, control, and artificial intelligence*. Cambridge, MA: CogNet. 1992.
3. Hansard. 18 May 1998, Column 1291. London: The Stationery Office.
4. Hawkes N. Children grow fatter as the experts dither. *The Times*, final edition 2006. London: *The Times*.
5. National Audit Office, Healthcare Commission and Audit Commission. Tackling Child Obesity – First Steps. HC801. London: The Stationery Office. 2006.
6. Plsek P.E., Greenhalgh T. Complexity science: the challenge of complexity in health care. *British Medical Journal* **323**: 625–628. 2001.
7. Wilson T., Holt T., Greenhalgh T. Complexity science: complexity and clinical care. *British Medical Journal* **323**: 685–688. 2001.
8. Plsek P.E., Wilson T. Complexity, leadership, and management in healthcare organisations. *British Medical Journal* **323**: 746–749. 2001.
9. Fraser S.W., Greenhalgh T. Coping with complexity: educating for capability. *British Medical Journal* **323**: 799–803. 2001.
10. Sweeney K., Griffiths F. *Complexity and Healthcare: An introduction*. Abingdon: Radcliffe Medical Press. 2002.
11. Kernick D. *Complexity and healthcare organization: A view from the street*. Abingdon: Radcliffe Medical Press. 2004.

12. Holt T.A. *Complexity for Clinicians*. Oxford: Radcliffe Medical Press. 2004.
13. Merali Y. Complexity and information systems. In: Social Theory and Philosophy for Information Systems (ed J. Mingers and L. Willcocks), pp.407–446. London: Wiley. 2004.
14. Caroll L. *Through the Looking Glass*.
15. Sturmberg J., Martin C., Moes M. Defining Health – A Dynamic Balance Model. 2006. Unpublished.
16. Fredriksen S. Instrumental colonisation in modern medicine. *Medical Health Care Philosophy* **6**: 287–296. 2003.
17. Idler E.L., Benyamini Y. Self-rated health and mortality: a review of twenty-seven community studies. *Journal of Health and Social Behavior* **38**: 21–37. 1997.
18. Glouberman S. Is there a health care system? A debate with Duncan Sinclair at Action Centre. http://www.healthandeverything.org/presentations/is_there_a_health_care_system.pdf. 2002. Accessed 15 April 2006.
19. Capra F. *The Web of Life: A new scientific understanding of living systems*. New York and London: Anchor Books. 1996.
20. Starfield B. *Primary Care: Balancing health needs, services, and technology*. New York and Oxford: Oxford University Press. 1998.
21. Innes A.D., Campion P.D., Griffiths F.E. Complex consultations and the 'edge of chaos'. *British Journal of General Practice* **55**: 47–52. 2005.
22. Innes A., Griffiths F., Campion P. Complexity and general practice: consulting at the 'edge of chaos'. *Family Practice* **22**: 91. 2005.
23. Kekki P. Primary Health Care and the Millenium Development Goals: Issues for Discussion. http://www.who.int/chronic_conditions/primary_health_care/en/mdgs_final.pdf. 2006. Accessed 26 March 2006.
24. Bortolotti M., Martin C. A theoretical Framework for Primary Health Care Transition. Ottawa, Canada: Virtual Office of Synthesis and Information. 2006.
25. Atun R.A. What are the advantages and disadvantages of restructuring a health care system to be more focused on primary care services? Imperial College, London Health Evidence Network (HEN), Director Health Management Programme, The Business School. 2006.
26. Keleher H. Why primary health care offers a more comprehensive approach to tackling health inequalities than primary care. *Australian Journal of Primary Care* **7**: 57–61. 2001.
27. Pan American Health Organization and World Health Organization. Regional Declaration on the new orientations for primary health care (Declaration of Montevideo). Washington, DC: Pan American Health Organization and World Health Organization. 2005.
28. Campbell S.M., Roland M.O., Middleton E. *et al*. Improvements in quality of clinical care in English general practice 1998–2003: longitudinal observational study. *British Medical Journal* **331**: 1121. 2005.
29. Smeeth L., Heath I. Why inequalities in health matter to primary care. *British Journal of General Practice* **51**: 436–437. 2001.
30. Smith P. On the unintended consequences of publishing performance data in the public sector. *International Journal of Public Administration* **18**: 277–310. 1995.
31. Huby G., Gerry M., McKinstry B. *et al*. Morale among general practitioners: qualitative study exploring relations between partnership arrangements, personal style, and workload. *British Medical Journal* **325**: 140. 2002.
32. Dershin H. Nonlinear systems theory in medical care management. *Physician Exectuives* **25**: 8–13. 1999.

33. Griffiths F., Byrne D. General practice and the new science emerging from the theories of 'chaos' and complexity. *British Journal of General Practice* **48**: 1697–1699. 1998.
34. Sweeney K., Griffiths F. *Complexity and Healthcare: An introduction.* Abingdon: Radcliffe Medical Press. 2002.
35. Dent E.B. Complexity science: a worldview shift. *Emergence* **1**: 5–19. 1999.
36. Miller W.L., Crabtree B.F., McDaniel R. *et al.* Understanding change in primary care practice using complexity theory. *Journal of Family Practice* **46**: 369–376. 1998.
37. Plsek P. Complexity and the adoption of innovation in health care (paper presentation). Washington DC: Conference on Accelerating Quality Improvement in Health Care. Conference proceeding. 2003.
38. Zimmerman B. Complexity science: a route through hard times and uncertainty. *Health Forum Journal* **42**: 42–46, 69. 1999.
39. Maniadakis N., Gray A. The economic burden of back pain in the UK. *Pain* **84**: 95–103. 2000.
40. Elliott A.M., Smith B.H., Penny K.I. *et al.* The epidemiology of chronic pain in the community. *The Lancet* **354**: 1248–1252. 1999.
41. Vrancken M.A. Schools of thought on pain. *Social Science and Medicine* **29**: 435–444. 1989.
42. Brown C.A. Service providers' perception of affective influences on decision-making about treatments for chronic pain. *Disability and Rehabilitation* **26**: 16–20. 2004.
43. Brown C. Consciousness, complexity and chronic pain: exploring the occurrence and implications of incongruent beliefs about 'important' chronic pain treatment components. University of Liverpool: Unpublished thesis. 2004.
44. Chew-Graham C.A., May C. 'Partners in pain' – the game of painmanship revisited. *Family Practice* **17**: 285–287. 2000.
45. Plsek P.E., Lindberg C., Zimmerman B. *Edgeware: Insights from complexity science for health care leaders.* Irving: VHA. 1998.
46. Gillespie R., Florin D., Gillam S. How is patient-centred care understood by the clinical, managerial and lay stakeholders responsible for promoting this agenda? *Health Expectations* **7**: 142–148. 2004.
47. Gordon D.B., Dahl J.L. Quality improvement challenges in pain management. *Pain* **107**: 1–4. 2004.
48. World Health Organization. World Health Report 2001: Mental Health, New Understanding, New Hope. Geneva: World Health Organization. 2001.
49. The Sainsbury Centre for Mental Health. *The economic and social costs of mental illness.* London: The Sainsbury Centre for Mental Health. 2003.
50. Weissman M.M., Bland R.C., Canino G.J. *et al.* The cross-national epidemiology of panic disorder. *Archives of General Psychiatry* **54**: 305–309. 1997.
51. Cilliers P. *Complexity and Postmodernism: Understanding complex systems.* London: Routledge. 1998.
52. Lambert R.A., Harvey I., Poland F. A pragmatic, unblinded randomised controlled trial comparing an occupational therapy-led lifestyle approach and routine GP care for panic disorder treatment in primary care. *J. Affect. Disord.* **99**: 63–71. 2007.
53. Denyer S.P., Stewart G.S.A.B. Mechanisms of action of disinfectants. *International Biodeterioration and biodegradation* **41**: 261–268. 1998.
54. Anonymous. European Suspension Test (1996): quantitative suspension test for the evaluation of the bactericidal activity of chemical disinfectants and antiseptics used in food, industrial, domestic and institutional areas. Test Method and requirements (Phase

2 step 1) prEN 1276 CEN/TC 216 N 109. European Committee for Standardisation. 1996.

55. Bloomfield S.F., Looney E. Evaluation of the repeatability and reproducibility of European suspension test methods for antimicrobial activity of disinfectants and antiseptics. *Journal of Applied Bacteriology* **73**: 87–93. 1992.

56. Bloomfield S.F., Arthur M., Van Klingeren B. *et al.* An evaluation of the repeatability and reproducibility of a surface test for the activity of disinfectants. *Journal of Applied Bacteriology* **76**: 86–94. 1994.

57. Rabone K.L., Rabone J.K., Rabone J.A.L. Simulation of disinfection using a cellular automata approach. 2006. In press.

58. Rachid F., Horobin R.W., Golding M.C.H.M. *et al.* Application of a simplistic Chinese-box model to the interaction of cultured cells with fluorescent probes. Institute of Physics Conference Series No. 98. 1998.

59. Vivaldi F. An experiment with mathematics. In: *New Scientist Guide to Chaos* (ed N. Hall). London: Penguin Science. 1991.

60. Agresti A. *An Introduction to Categorical Data Analysis.* New York: Wiley. 1996.

61. Watson M.J. Do patients with severe traumatic brain injury benefit from physiotherapy? A review of the evidence. *Physical Therapy Reviews* **6**: 233–249. 2001.

62. Gracies J.M., Marosszeky J.E., Renton R. *et al.* Short-term effects of dynamic lycra splints on upper limb in hemiplegic patients. *Archives of Physical Medicine and Rehabilitation* **81**: 1547–1555. 2000.

63. Watson M., Horn S. 'The ten pound note test': suggestions for eliciting improved responses in the severely brain-injured patient. *Brain Injury* **5**: 421–424. 1991.

64. Watson M.J., Hitchcock R. Recovery of walking late after a severe traumatic brain injury. *Physiotherapy* **90**: 103–107. 2004.

65. Mengshoel A.M. Physiotherapy and the placebo effect. *Physical Therapy Reviews* **5**: 161–165. 2000.

66. Arup. The Millennium Bridge. http://www.arup.com/MillenniumBridge/. 2006.

67. Bullock S., Cliff D., Ince M. *Complexity and Emergent Behaviour in Information and Communications Systems.* 2004. London: UK Department of Trade and Industry Foresight Directorate.

68. Waldrop M.M. *Complexity: The emerging science at the edge of order and chaos.* Harmondsworth: Penguin Books. 1994.

69. Wikipedia. Homeostasis. http://en.wikipedia.org/wiki/homeostasis. 2006.

70. Jones G.R., Russell P.C., Vourdas A. *et al.* The Gabor transform basis of chromatic monitoring. *Measurement Science & Technology* **11**: 489–498. 2000.

71. Deakin A.G., Rallis I., Zhang J. *et al.* Towards holistic chromatic intelligent monitoring of complex systems. International Complexity Science & Society Conference, University of Liverpool. 11 September 2005.

72. Rallis I., Deakin A.G., Spencer J.W. *et al.* Novel sensing techniques for industrial scale bio-digesters. Voet Marc, Willsch, Reinhardt, Ecke, Wolfgang, Jones, Julian, and Culshaw, Brian. 2005. SPIE Volume 5855, 17th International Conference on Optical Fibre Sensors.

73. MIMS Project Manager. Merton Intelligent Monitoring System (MIMS). http://www.merton.gov.uk/living/health/mims.htm. 2005.

74. Deakin A.G., Spencer J.W., Jones G.R. A chromatic approach to complexity. International Complexity Science and Society Conference, University of Liverpool. Conference proceeding. 2005.

75. Wong K.J., Xu S., Jones G.R. Chromatic identification of complex movement patterns. In: *Proceedings of the Complex Systems Monitoring Session of the International Complexity Science and Society Conference*, CIMS, Liverpool. 2005, pp.24–28.

76. Russell C.D., Deakin A.G., Jones G.R. Chromatic analysis for signal processing in optical coherence tomography. In: *Proceedings of the Complex Systems Monitoring Session of the International Complexity Science and Society Conference*, CIMS, Liverpool. 2005, pp.40–45.

77. Rallis I., Glomon L., Deakin A.G. *et al.* Polychromatic monitoring of complex biological factors. In: *Proceedings of the Complex Systems Monitoring Session of the International Complexity Science and Society Conference*, CIMS, Liverpool. 2005, pp.40–45.

78. Zhang J., Jones G.R. Chromatic processing for event probability description. In: *Proceedings of the Complex Systems Monitoring Session of the International Complexity Science and Society Conference*, CIMS, Liverpool. 2005, pp.61–67.

79. Kolupula Y.R., Reichelt T.E., Aceves Fernandez M.A. *et al.* Chromatic methodologies for information extraction from complex data sets. In: *Proceedings of the Complex Systems Monitoring Session of the International Complexity Science and Society Conference*, CIMS, Liverpool. 2005, pp.68–76.

80. Costa M., Goldberger A.L., Peng C.-K. Multiscale entropy analysis of complex physiologic time series. *Physical Review Letters* **89**: 068102. 2002.

81. Holt T.A. A chaotic model for tight diabetes control. *Diabetic Medicine* **19**: 274–278. 2002.

82. Kaplan D., Glass L. *Understanding Nonlinear Dynamics*, pp.308–311. New York: Springer-Verlag. 1995.

CHAPTER 6

International relations and development

Edited by Robert Geyer

Introduction

Strange as this may seem, given that the international system and development must be among the most complex social processes that can be studied, academics and policy actors spent most of the latter half of the 20th century feverishly trying to prove that they were fundamentally simple and orderly. Particularly during the apparent bi-polar simplicity of the Cold War, international relations experts produced a plethora of quantitative studies emphasising linear modelling methods that tried to explore the conditions and likelihood of war and revolution. Early critics noted that, though statistically elegant, these studies were not particularly good at predicting, yet alone reflecting, reality. Despite these criticisms, these efforts continued and it was hoped that greater computer power would solve the problem. It did offer a range of new tools, but the emphasis on fundamental order and the division within the field between more modernist and postmodernist interpretations remains as strong as ever.

Likewise, international economic development theory went through a similar process. Pressured by the political needs of the Cold War, rapid economic development of the, so-called, Third World was seen as being essential to the future of the, so-called, West. Clear pathways and policies were laid out based on the already successful Western model. Development was just a matter of effort and following the right path. Despite the clear failure of the early modernisation theories, the belief that there was one fundamental approach to development continued and rapidly expanded with the emergence of the 'debt crisis', and the consequent creation of the linear and orderly Structural Adjustment Policies of the World Bank/Inetrnational Monetary Fund. The deepening of the debt crisis and failure of the adjustment policies has led to a continual process of revision and crisis in development thinking.

In both international relations and development thinking the time is ripe for complexity. In international relations, edited books exploring the implications of complexity are starting to emerge such as Edgar Grande and Louis Pauly (editors) *Complex Sovereignty* [1], and Neil Harrison (editor) *Complexity and World Politics* [2]. Meanwhile, in development theory, Samir Rihani's seminal work, *Complex Systems Theory and Development Practice* [3], is already starting to have a noticeable impact on the field.

This chapter will introduce some of the new work in these burgeoning fields. To begin, Kai Lehmann provides a fascinating study of the process of political decision-making centralisation in the aftermath of the events of 11 September. He argues that this process is founded on a traditional orderly view of politics and society and, using complexity, he not only challenges the need to centralise decision-making in the aftermath of international 'shock' events, but argues that centralisation is only capable of dealing with simple shocks and cannot handle more complex situations such as the so-called 'war on terror'. In the following section, Abbie Badcock, building on Rihani's pathbreaking work, argues that despite unprecedented economic resources and intellectual efforts, the universal 'one-size-fits-all' linear approach to development theory of the post-World War II period has not accelerated the 'catch-up' process or even narrowed the economic gap between the First and Third Worlds. Using a complexity framework, argues Badcock, is the only way of recognising the true diversity of development and small but fundamental steps that individual countries must take to find their own way forward and truly develop.

Applying complexity to international affairs: 11 September and the war on terrorism
Kai Lehmann

Introduction

The terrorist attacks of 11 September 2001 have been seen by many as world-changing events, a view that was advanced by both academics and politicians [4–6]. However, the political response to these events was utterly predictable: President Bush, for instance, saw 11 September as attacks on 'freedom and democracy' and declared them to be 'acts of war' [7]. To deal with this threat, he subsequently declared a 'war on terrorism' which 'will not end until every terrorist group of global reach has been found, stopped and defeated' [8]. As a consequence, policy decision-making power centralised around the Executive and in particular the President, as it has done traditionally in times of crisis[1].

Having briefly traced the process leading up to a declaration of a war on terrorism, the rest of this section will be dedicated to challenging the concept of a war on terrorism. In doing so, I will argue that the concept of a 'war' and the centralisation of power this brings with it does not do justice to the complexities involved in dealing with the issue of terrorism. I will propose that, rather than seeing terrorism as a linear concept that can be defeated by conducting a war, one should conceptualise it as a complex adaptive system. This will not only help in understanding the phenomenon of terrorism better, but also in managing expectations of 'success' in dealing with the problem. As such, the application of complexity will help avoid some of the most extreme, unhelpful and indeed counterproductive measures taken in order to win a 'war' which, in reality, has no

---

1 This centralisation is based on the constitution. Article 2 of the American constitution allows the President extensive powers in times of national emergencies that are time-limited. The idea that power should centralise around the leader of the Executive in times of crisis is very old. Machiavelli, Hobbes and Locke, for instance, all argued that states need a strong leader to deal with crises [9–11]. An extensive literature exists debating whether 11 September constitutes such an emergency [12–14].

realistic chance of success. Finally, therefore, complexity theory will be used to establish realistic targets to deal with the threat of terrorism.

Linearity, centralisation and the war on terrorism

The process of centralisation that followed the attacks of 11 September was incredibly quick. Having declared the attacks 'acts of war' on 12 September, Bush then declared a national emergency on 14 September [15][2]. Congress subsequently granted the president authority to use military force[3]. With his speech of 20 September specifically setting out a war on terrorism, it only took 10 days for Bush to have all the legal and political authority to frame the US response any way he saw fit and on his terms[4]. Essentially, therefore, the terms of the 'war on terrorism' were framed by him. These terms can be summarised as follows:

- The war on terror was to be an all-encompassing war with no room for compromise.

  As Bush himself put it on 20 September:

  > 'Every nation, in every region, now has a decision to make. Either you are with us or you are with the terrorists. From this day forward, any nation that continues to harbour or support terrorism will be regarded by the United States as a hostile regime' [8].

- The war on terrorism could therefore be fought against clearly identifiable targets. This was further underlined when Bush constructed an 'axis of evil' in his State of the Union Address of 2002, comprising those countries he claimed were actively supporting terrorist activity [17][5].
- The war on terrorism would be fought pro-actively, if necessary through pre-emptive attacks [18].
- The war on terrorism would be won by promoting active American leadership across the globe, instigating regime change where needed and promoting liberal democratic principles[6].

In many ways, therefore, the response to 11 September was stunningly simple: following the above steps would lead to a 'victory' in the war on terrorism and hence make the United States a safer place.

Yet, such simplicity masked some serious problems inherent in the concept, which many commentators soon picked up on.

The key problem surely with declaring a war on terrorism is the fact that no-one is quite sure what one is actually fighting. There simply is no agreed definition of the term [20–22]. As such, it is a mistake to try to '*isolate a single phenomena labelled "terrorism"*' [22: p.197]. In fact, it will make it harder to deal with the problem. Bearing in mind the problem of definition, there is virtually no chance of eradicating terrorism.

---

2 Under the National Emergencies Act of 1976, such a declaration activates almost 160 provisions of law.
3 Public Law 107-40 was enacted to enable this authority.
4 For a detailed account of the reaction of Bush's inner circle, see [16].
5 The 'axis of evil' included Iraq, Iran and North Korea.
6 This is the so-called 'Bush doctrine', as summarised by Schmitt and Donnelly [19].

A second problem with the concept of a war on terrorism is its total emphasis on security, which focuses the response on the traditional means of security policy, i.e. the military. This focus is too narrow: *'Military might without a vision for which it should be used might ensure short-term gains, [but] it would not be sufficient in combating terrorism'* [23: p.294].

Of course, the Bush administration would deny that it did not have a vision. Bush has expressed a clear commitment to the spread of liberal democracy and all this would entail, including respect for human rights, and the protection of individual freedoms[7]. Yet, the experience in both Afghanistan and Iraq seems to suggest that such a universally accepted model for society does not exist. Indeed, experience shows that parts of the world actively resist such a vision, seeing it as a *Western* concept that has to be resisted, particularly when such a concept is *imposed* rather than *offered*.

The common theme here, then, seems to be that the war on terrorism is a linear concept that assumes that there is *one* way to deal with terrorism, and in which various authoritarian and dictatorial regimes can be replaced by *one* model of societal organisation, i.e. an American version of liberal democracy. Unfortunately, the consequences of such linearity are all too obvious.

Fundamentally, the war on terrorism has failed to achieve its objective of defeating terrorism. In fact, the opposite has occurred. According to the State Department, there were 651 'significant' terrorist attacks in the year 2004, compared with 175 in the year 2003. In those attacks, 1907 people were killed, compared with 625 the year before [24]. The consequences of this approach, however, go far deeper than 'merely' an increase in terrorist activity. As Gaddis has observed, such a simplistic approach to terrorism has led to a situation where *'[f]rom nearly universal sympathy in the weeks after September 11, Americans within a year and a half found their country widely regarded as an international pariah'* [25: p.6]. The simple fact is that *'using massive military force against terrorism…tends to create more terrorists'* [26: p.276]. The very predictability and certainty of outcome that the 'war' on terrorism was meant to provide has instead led to a situation in which the world is now a far more radicalised place than it had been previously. The linear approach has fundamentally failed in achieving its objectives. It is at this point that complexity theory can help.

Terrorism as a complex adaptive system

Terrorism can clearly be seen as a complex adaptive system:
- it has numerous internal elements;
- it is governed by local interactions between those numerous internal elements;
- the system is maintained by exchanging energies with other systems;
- the system is capable of evolving [27].

Terrorism, just like other complex systems, is characterised by its excessive diversity and its incompressibility. That is to say, any description of it must be necessarily incomplete or else be as complex as the system itself. Such recognition has serious implications for the impact any policy can have in dealing with the problem. As such, policy makers have to recognise that:

---

7 The National Security Strategy of 2002 speaks of a 'single sustainable model for national success' that is 'right and true for every person in every society' [18].

- the state can expect to do little more than to create a stable framework within which individuals can maximise their potential through interaction[8];
- a recognition of complexity should lead to a more open, pluralistic policy-making framework. The more complex the policy-making environment, the more flexible the policies and the better the chances for adjustments, thereby avoiding mistakes;
- policy making should be evolutionary and be based on successive adjustments.

The above suggests that the policy-making process is a messy, sometimes even an incomprehensible affair in which rationality is important, while at the same time being tempered by any number of other factors that will play into the decision-making process. From a traditional social science point of view, this is a problem. It surely cannot be good not to know. However, from a complexity point of view, a 'messy' and complex policy process is not only inevitable, but it is actually a good thing and is to be encouraged. It is this very complexity which keeps most political systems afloat. Excessive order, the imposition of restrictive frameworks on countries, populations or indeed academics, is not only stifling but counterproductive [28].

What does all this mean for the approach to dealing with terrorism? I believe the key is to recognise that there will not be a single solution to the problem. A war on such a multi-faceted concept, fought through a command and control structure, has as much chance of success as the much-trumpeted war on drugs, i.e. none. Take for instance the current focus on Islamic terrorism. As has been demonstrated elsewhere, in statistical terms this is the wrong focus to start with because, for most of the previous decades, terrorist attacks were primarily against US business interests in Latin America, not the Middle East [28]. However, even if Islamic terrorism *was* correctly the main focus of attention, we would still be dealing with 'a hugely varied and shifting phenomena' [29: p.15].

If the question of fighting terrorism *was* a simple question of 'taking out' known terrorists and destroying terrorist infrastructure, then one could argue that there have been significant successes. Since 2001, 'two thirds of the Al Quaeda "leadership" has been eliminated one way or another' [29: p.260]. In addition, the base for its operations in Afghanistan has been destroyed, forcing most operatives to flee and scatter. As such, one would expect Islamic terrorism to be less of a problem now than it may have been in 2001. However, the evidence suggests that the opposite is the case. As Jason Burke has pointed out:

> *'The world is a far more radicalised place now than it was before 11 September. Helped by a powerful surge of anti-Americanism, by Washington's incredible failure to stem the haemorrhaging of support and sympathy, and by modern communications, the language of bin Laden and his concept of cosmic struggle has now spread among tens of millions of people, particularly the young and angry, around the world'* [29: p.274].

---

8 The state may be able to affect change, but it is not able to control long-term developments. So, for our purposes, governments may be able to round-up and convict terrorists in the short term, but they are not able to guarantee the eradication of terrorism in the long term.

Far from dealing with terrorism, the 'war' on the phenomenon has given many radical leaders in the Islamic world the very 'cosmic struggle' they have always sought.

What though could be done instead? The following steps may be useful. First, responsibility for fighting terrorism needs to be decentralised. Iraqis, for example, should be left in charge of their own affairs to deal with the 'insurgency'. This is doubly important because some of the current terrorist activity may spring from resentment to the very concepts that we in the West see as the best guarantor to defeat terrorism, i.e. liberal democracy and a free-market economy. As Rihani points out: *'Foreigners [...] do not hate America or the Americans. They hate the corporate powers that masquerade as "the USA" and seek under that banner to dominate whole nations in the name of freedom and democracy'* [30]. What this suggests is that to deal with the issue of terrorism requires tackling deep-seated misgivings about a broad range of issues in large parts of the world, especially the idea that there is one 'right' way to organise a society, which is a Western-style liberal democracy, underpinned by a neo-liberal, free-market economy.

This, of course, is not the case. We need to acknowledge that what we have grown used to is not necessarily the best for others. In fact, we need to acknowledge that for much of history the current established capitalist, liberal-democratic states have evolved: the USA did not begin to truly open herself up to the world economy until the beginning of the 20th century. In Western Europe, countries such as West Germany and France derived much of their economic strength and stability from having extensive welfare provisions.

Crucially, they were allowed to get on with it in their own way[9]. Western countries, therefore, thrive as complex adaptive systems, which allow the political system enough flexibility to adjust to changing circumstances and demands. A similar approach should be taken in relation to international politics and the war on terror.

There also needs to be some honesty. In the aftermath of the terrorist attacks in London in July 2005, Tony Blair rightly pointed out that there is no such thing as absolute security and that an 'open' society will have to live with the risk. Yet, the same Prime Minister also signed up to the 'war' on terror, vowing to 'defeat' the terrorists, and has argued enthusiastically for the war in Iraq as part of this wider struggle [27][10]. Yet, his Home Secretary proposes to store private e-mails as part of the war on terror even though there is no evidence that this would significantly deter terrorists.

Contrast this with Tony Blair's approach to the Northern Ireland conflict and compare the result. If flexibility is required to deal with Northern Irish terrorists, how much more is required to deal with the problem as a whole?

George Bush has shown similar inconsistencies. On the one hand, one of his first acts in his second term was to appoint Barbara Hughes as Undersecretary of State to re-engage the USA with international partners. On the other, he sees the attacks in London as further evidence that the war on terrorism must continue in its current

---

9 On the importance of this see Gaddis [31].

10 See for instance the Prime Minister's speech in the House of Commons opening the Iraq debate on 18 March 2003 [32].

form [33]. We therefore find ourselves in the bizarre situation where leaders, policy makers and commentators clearly recognise the fact that a 'war' on terrorism is not going to plan and yet are unwilling or unable to change policy. To deal with this problem we have to keep asking 'why' and we need to be flexible.

Conclusion

This section has shown that the 'war on terrorism' is a typical way of responding to major political crises. It reflects the well-established linear framework within which most states conduct crisis management. I have argued that this approach has patently failed to tackle terrorism and has indeed made the problem worse than it was before.

To more effectively deal with the issue of terrorism I have argued that we should conceive of it as a 'complex adaptive system' with indefinite and indeterminate causes, many of which will remain unknown to us. Such a re-conceptualisation would require policy makers to broaden their framework of analysis and to honestly acknowledge their chances of success in dealing with the problem. This may be uncomfortable, but it is necessary. It will force policy makers to open up the policy process, adopt more flexible policy-responses and deal with the possibility of failure.

Such an undertaking would have avoided many of the problems we are experiencing in places such as Iraq. It may well have led to a different policy decision in relation to this conflict. Even if it had not, admissions of fallibility and corrections of policy would make the 'coalition forces' appear more humble and therefore perhaps result in a softening of attitudes.

Complexity theory therefore acknowledges that there may not be a solution to every problem. Governments may just be able to effect short-term changes, but they can in no way guarantee, for instance, the success of a democratic Iraq or the defeat of terrorism. In fact, any such proclamation would be dishonest. To avoid the most severe consequences of making mistakes, the policy process needs to be as open as possible as often as possible. Interaction leads to policy innovation, recognition of errors and therefore helps to avoid crises in the first place. This is crucial because, as Rihani points out:

> 'The affairs of humankind, from individuals to the whole global community, unfold along an uncertain, evolutionary path that could not be directed by commands from the top. Changes take time, links between causes and effects are not readily obvious, trial and error and copious diversity are at a premium, and outcomes are full of surprises' [30].

To achieve a situation where this is readily accepted will take not only a lot of persuasion but also a lot of further research, especially on the question of how the policy-making process can be reformed to take account of the insights from complexity. However, the mess that has become the war on terrorism and the enormous human costs this has brought in its wake suggest that this undertaking would not only be time well spent, but that it is also an urgent thing to do.

Can complexity save development theory?

Abbie Badcock

Introduction

Despite huge efforts, billions of dollars and the occasional rock concert (LiveAid in the 1980s and Live8 in 2005), the limited results of development strategies, mixed at best catastrophic at worst, have been a cause of continual frustration to policy practitioners and academics (let alone the people living in the so-called Developing World). In the mid-1990s a major UNDP document reported that, *'no fewer than 100 countries − all developing or in transition − have experience[d] serious economic decline over the past three decades. As a result, per capita income in these 100 countries is lower than it was 10, 20, even 30 years ago'* [34: p.37]. The most recent UNDP report paints a similar picture: *'In 2003, 18 countries with a combined population of 460 million people registered lower scores on the human development index (HDI) than in 1990 − an unprecedented reversal'* [35: p.3].

What is going wrong? Is it too much or too little markets, state action, aid, external interference, policy knowledge, etc.? Moreover, what can be done about it? In this brief section, following in the footsteps of Samir Rihani and his groundbreaking book *Complex Systems Theory and Development Practice* [3], we argue that the failing of dominant traditional theories of development (modernisation, structural adjustment, etc.) is because they are based within a fundamentally 'linear' framework which assumes that:

- there is just one path or line of true development;
- this path has a stable and achievable endpoint (to emulate existing 'developed' nations);
- individual nations can be positioned along this pathway and appropriate policy strategies can be developed by knowledgeable elites;
- 'top-down' models of development can deliver calculated and measurable results.

However, as made clear by the UN documents mentioned above, widespread success has not occurred, and the universal 'one-size-fits-all' linear approach to development theory has not accelerated the 'catch-up' process or even narrowed the economic gap between the First and Third Worlds. Obviously, there are many competing theories to the dominant linear ones: Basic Needs, Dependency, NIEO, Sustainable Development and Underdevelopment, to name just a few. Over time, these have risen and fallen with different historical events and academic and policy actors. What these theories have failed to do is confront the scientific foundation of the dominant linear approach, and have always appeared to be weaker, softer and less certain than the more 'scientific' dominant theories.

Complexity is different. Emerging out of the physical sciences in the 20th century and spilling over into the social sciences and public policy in the 21st, it directly challenges the fundamental framework of linear theories by postulating a new scientific paradigm. This framework argues that the natural and human worlds combine order and disorder, certainty and uncertainty and predictability and unpredictability, in an emergent complex adaptive system that does not conform to rigid universal laws, rules or policy proscriptions.

The remainder of this section will briefly outline why and how the linear concept of development emerged and what complexity offers as an alternative.

The linearity of traditional development theory

To understand how traditional development theory became synonymous with a linear mindset, it is necessary to look back to the development of modern academia. Sir Isaac Newton's discovery of the laws of gravity gave hope to theorists that we, as humans, are able to know and therefore determine the laws of the universe and apply them to the social and physical sciences [36: p.21]. Knowledge is finite and could rationalise the disorderly and uncertain, whilst scientific studies could be used to predict and determine knowable causes that would result in certain effects. The structural framework or paradigm from this point onwards was locked into the idea that effects could be determined, problems could be managed and understood through reductionism, and outcomes could therefore be predicted [37: p.19].

In the field of development studies, the consequences of this paradigm had similar implications for both the political left and right. For example, in the 19th century Karl Marx conceived his historical and theoretical analysis of the capitalist modes of production and development as a line of stages that needed to be fulfilled to arrive at a communist endpoint [38, 39]. Likewise, but on the Right, Walt Rostow in the mid-20th century developed the anti-communist 'modernisation theory' that described the five stages of growth from 'the traditional society' to 'the age of high mass-consumption'. Even his concept of 'traditional society' was based on a linear approach of a 'pre-Newtonion science', and in his own words, Newton was seen as a:

> 'watershed in history when men came widely to believe that the external world was subject to few knowable laws, and was systematically capable of productive manipulation' [40: p.100].

This concept of developmental linearity can also be visualised on an *X–Y* axis, where the level of development will increase over time (see Figure 6.1) – the idea being that all countries were travelling along the same line. The focus of modernisation was to get them further up the line as fast as possible and ideally, from Rostow's perspective, integrated into the Western bloc.

Rostow's work has to be viewed in relation to its historical setting. During the de-colonisation period of the late 1940s and early 1950s, the onset of the Cold War played a significant threat and encouraged the USA to actively campaign for Third World economic development, with the desire of marginalising the number of

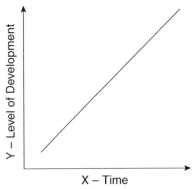

Figure 6.1. A linear visualisation of traditional development.

communist supporters or 'bedfellows'. Later, the 'Washington Consensus' built upon the foundation of modernisation theory and, using the lever of the growing Third World debt crisis, soon dominated development thinking. This new consensus, with its top-down model guidelines set by the International Monetary Fund (IMF) and World Bank, and a belief that the formula of free international trade and open markets could be universally applied to accelerate the development process, has dominated development thinking to the present day. In this context, developed countries were goals at the finishing line of the development scale and highly educated economists would provide the guidance to encourage lesser developed countries to 'catch up'. McMichael notes that:

> *'Developmentalism... was a constructed order [of] ... evolutionary progression along a linear trajectory of modernization. In this respect, not only would each state replicate the modernity of the First World, but there were expectations that the development gap between First and Third Worlds would be progressively closed'* [41: p.278].

Underdeveloped states were viewed as backward and required external intervention, with the underlying assumption *'that the Western lifestyle and mode of economic organisation were superior and should be universally aspired to'* [42: p.564]. Industrialisation was to be the first step and developing countries were unlikely to protest to this opportunity of joining the 'First World Club'. States were expected to replicate the development project *'that was a view of [artificially] ordering the world'* [41: p.279]. With regards to developmentalism in follower countries, it was thought that:

> *'if they follow the leading countries' pattern of development, countries attempting to take off toward industrialization will readily see which industries to introduce and how rapidly and in what order they should import technologies'* [43: p.303].

The modernisation process would not guarantee equality, but an economic 'trickle-down effect' would help to deliver better living standards and in turn narrow the economic gap between First and Third World countries. Full implementation of IMF and World Bank policies would be beneficial to all. A huge influx of foreign aid flooded the developing world as the IMF and World Bank were keen to lend their support. However, the OPEC-initiated 'oil crises' during the 1970s, growing international interest rates, increasing First World protectionism and declining commodity prices had serious ramifications for developing countries. The UN's agencies, and in particular the USA, recalled their financial loans and demanded repayments to start. Unsurprisingly, the money had gone, with little to show for it and no means of repayment. Specialisation and mono-crop production not only led to economic failure within the international system for developing countries, but also resulted in worse living standards than under colonial rule. Not only did the conditions worsen, but rapid Latin American growth was arrested by the debt crisis, and only the industrialising East Asian countries were able to weather the storm [38: p.301].

East Asian countries, considered to be further along the 'developmental scale', were able to *adapt* the economic policies to suit their own economies and by doing so protect their own interests. This adaptation is exactly what complexity deems necessary for a system to survive under harsh conditions. Following in the footsteps of Japan's economic development, ' ... *the "four dragons" of East Asia [Taiwan, Korea, Singapore and Hong Kong], succeeded in the takeoff [of economic growth] by adapting the developmentalist model to their own economies*' [43: p.303].

But with regards to the unsuccessful developing countries, the experts working in the Washington consensus agreed that because the model was correct it must be the fault of internal weaknesses such as corrupt governments, overburdening state, mismanagement of modernisation policies, over reliance on foreign aid/ loans, or a range of other national frailties. It was just strange that so many countries could get it so wrong, so often.

Complexity theory, however, would argue that the problem was not with the countries, but with the rigidity and linearity of the model. For complexity, a universal model for all countries could never work, especially if it does not allow for local variety and interpretation. Rigid linear models rested on the notion that effects could be reliably predicted. In reality, probable effects can only be contemplated. Positive or negative feedback may exaggerate a situation, causing what Lorenz described as a 'Butterfly effect', whereby a small cause could have an unforeseen effect [44: pp.6–20]. For example, a *'given cause might lead to more than one outcome, and if the process were repeated the results could be, and often are, different*' [45: p.239]. This relationship and interaction between elements can be described as a complex relationship.

Essentially, development is not a simple or even complicated problem but a complex one, and as such simple or complicated 'solutions' (look at some of the enormous UN documents on development), regardless of whether intentions are altruistic or not, will not be able to adequately deal with the issue.

Time for a new paradigm shift?

As described by Rihani [46], development theory has already started a shift towards alternative approaches. In his pathbreaking and impressively engaging work, Rihani endeavours to convince the reader that scholars need to adopt a very different framework of assessment when viewing the concept of development. In this perspective, nations must be understood as 'complex adaptive systems' and, as a consequence, development has 'no beginning, no end point and no short-cuts' [3]. Development is always slow, uneven and open-ended.

Complexity theory offers a significant re-conceptualisation of how one perceives the developmental process. All countries, regardless of their current economic status, have undergone a long and lengthy process of evolution. This process can be steady, but also unexpectedly rapid at times, and exhibit what some authors have termed 'punctuated equilibrium' [47: pp.98–100]. For example, Britain underwent rapid change and development after the onset of the Industrial Revolution in the 19th century, followed by later periods of stability and stagnation.

A period of relative calm (perceived as order) will occur in the international system, usually centred around a stabilising force (or 'attractor'). The bi-polar era during the Cold War had two stabilising attractors, each undergoing its own development. This process, similar to hegemonic stability theory, is cyclical, and small causes in the system can intensify due to positive and negative feedback, causing an attractor to change and therefore punctuate the period of 'equilibrium'. The swift and non-violent end of Soviet communism seemed to happen instantly, but was the culmination of negative feedback over a long period of time[11]. Simple causality, therefore, does not always apply to complex systems.

But what does this have to do with development theory? The acknowledgement of this lengthy process allows the observer to realise the limitations of aspiring to an ideal endpoint in development. Complexity views development as '*not a rush to the nearest summit but a leisurely process of exploration of possibilities*' [45: p.240]. One way of visualising this exploratory process is through the concept of a fitness landscape (Figure 6.2) rather than the linearity of the *X–Y* graph.

With the concept of a fitness landscape, exploration of all the options available is just as important as reaching the summit. For a complex system to be able to develop, diversity and local interactions need to *emerge* and can be described as *emergent properties*, which did not exist previously and could not be forced upon the system from a top-down model or by external intervention.

Complex adaptive systems are comprised of many internal elements. The numerous elements must be permitted to interact with one another at the local level. Local interactions are extremely important and described as being '*dynamic*' as they exhibit global patterns of behaviour. These patterns of activity will '*acquire self-organized stable patterns ... as the cumulative outcomes from local interactions between internal elements of the system*' [48: p.134]. Interactions have to be regulated by simple rules to prevent chaos and allow global patterns to emerge. These rules cannot be so rigid or oppressive that they prevent the system from being able to adapt and evolve by enforcing an unnatural structure upon society.

The development of each nation, therefore, needs to be allowed to evolve independently of repressive authoritarian governments or excessive external interference that can stifle local interactions, diversity and self-organisation. Similarly, a nation needs to have an infrastructure whereby the general populous can follow simple, but non-intrusive rules, to allow this self-organisation to develop.

It is therefore within these two boundaries of stifling order and anarchic chaos that successful complex adaptive systems can develop. With Western development, every state has evolved and emerged as unique and individual. Each developed country has diversified and adapted to its own assets, and interprets concepts like 'democracy' and 'identity' differently.

These conditions allow for the successful development of countries and what we see is a tendency for complexity in society to increase. The 'gap' therefore between developed and underdeveloped countries cannot and will not be rapidly decreased. Economic measures or statistics do not highlight an individual nation-state's development subject to its own challenges or cumulated history. It would be worthwhile to recognise the difference between developing and non-developing areas and to realise the opportunities and capabilities that these regions have, rather than enforce them to conform to a particular model (such as the 'specialisation' tactics of Ricardian comparative advantage mono-crops). More localised measures would help generate greater interactions and boost the economic system.

---

11 This event can also be described as a 'gateway event' that opened up a new cascade of potential possibilities for ex-communist states to develop.

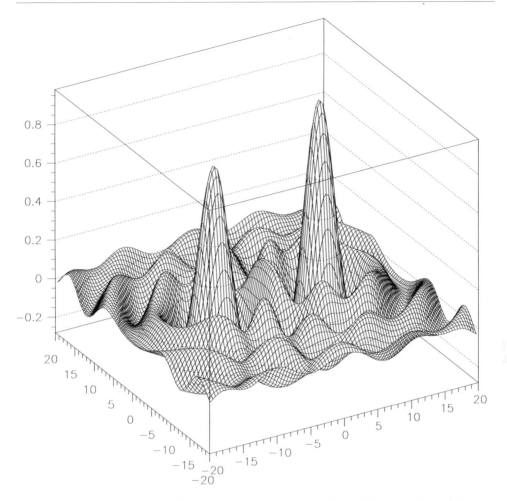

Figure 6.2. Fitness landscape available at www.talkorigins.org/design/fags/nfl/ (accessed January 2007).

What are the implications of complexity for development theory?

Complexity conceptualises development as a multi-faceted, nonlinear, adaptive and ongoing process. Subsequently, hierarchical or centralised strategies of development that do not emerge from local interactions and activity will not result in successful results. Development needs to diversify at the local level to enable interactions to flourish and emerge. The European Union as a governing and sponsorship body for the progress of underdeveloped European countries has looked to specifically target local regions to address this problem, and draw upon the ideas of sustainable rather than purely economic growth.

In addition, development strategy needs to include *human* development. Both Rihani and Geyer [45: p.244] note that a shift in focus needs to be adopted to incorporate *'improving standards of health, nutrition, literacy, democracy and governance'*, and that *'without decisive actions to address these fundamental issues the process of development [cannot] begin.'* Rihani adds that:

'[c]urrent development efforts are founded on an implicit belief that benefits from economic development will trickle down to uplift the fortunes of most members of the population. A view of development founded on complexity would turn that argument on its head. It maintains that no development is possible unless most members of the population are in a position to drive that effort forward' [48: p.139].

Local knowledge specific to individual localities, regions and countries can assist in enabling greater diversity and interaction to develop, but must adopt a decentralised grass-roots approach to warrant any validity in the development process. A large variety of inputs and outputs need to be incorporated into the system to enable it to self-organise and adapt, ensuring resistance to future situations that might de-stabilise the structure. The East-Asian Tiger countries succumbed to massive financial setbacks following economic crisis in the late 1990s. Even though they suffered financially, the structure did not collapse due to the extensive layers of complexity that had been developed during their growth periods. They were able to realign themselves and adapt to economic pressures without societal collapse. For this reason, the IMF is increasingly acknowledging the need to adopt medium- and long-term strategies with flexibility to adapt to changes in circumstances. It also acknowledges the limitations to their projections.

Complexity: the development saviour?

The linear models of traditional development theory, epitomised by Karl Marx's 'capitalist mode of production', Rostow's 'Five stages of economic growth' and Washington consensus, perceive progress as a smooth line or escalator of economic growth. Complexity provides a scientific framework for a much more open-minded approach to an ongoing and open-ended process. Fundamentally, complex systems cannot be determined, predicted or reduced into component parts, and will appear chaotic at the local level but emit general patterns at the global.

There can be no single 'universal' law of development, as every developed country has undergone its own distinctive process of evolution. Diversity and uniqueness are assets in complex systems as they are able to develop and adapt to changes in their local and global environment, thereby making them stronger systems in the long term. A more decentralised approach needs to be taken to allow complexity to emerge under suitable conditions. Simple rules must exist that are non-intrusive to prevent the system falling into too much order or chaos.

Finally, though he does not come out of a complexity framework, I feel that Lawrence Harrison [49: p.2] best describes the complexity interpretation of development theory when he states that:

'the creative capacity of human beings is at the heart of the development process. What makes development happen is our ability to imagine, theorize, conceptualize, experiment, invent, articulate, organize, to imagine, solve problems, and do a hundred other things with our minds and hands that contribute to the progress of the individual and of human-kind.'

References

1. Grande E., Pauly L. *Complex Sovereignty: Reconstituting political authority in the twenty-first century.* Toronto: University of Toronto Press. 2005.
2. Harrison N. *Complexity and World Politics: Concepts and methods of a new paradigm.* New York: State University of New York Press. 2006.
3. Rihani S. *Complex Systems Theory and Development Practice.* London: Zed Books. 2002.
4. Runciman D. A bear armed with a gun. *London Review of Books* **25** (7). 2003.
5. Halliday F. *Two Hours That Shook the World: September 11, 2001 – Causes and consequences.* London: Saqi Books. 2001.
6. Kagan R. *Of Paradise and Power – America and Europe in the New World Order.* London: Atlantic Books. 2003.
7. Bush G.W. Remarks by the President in Photo Opportunity with the National Security Team, Office of the Press Secretary, The White House. 12 September 2001 (accessed via www.whitehouse.gov).
8. Bush G.W. Address to a Joint Session of Congress and the American People. Office of the Press Secretary, The White House. 20 September 2001(b) (accessed via www.whitehouse.gov).
9. Skinner Q. *Visions of Politics – Volume 2: Renaissance virtues.* Cambridge: Cambridge University Press. 2002.
10. Boucher D., Kelly P. (editors). *Political Thinkers – From Socrates to the present.* Oxford: Oxford University Press. 2003.
11. Rossiter C.L. *Constitutional Dictatorship – Crisis government in the modern democracies.* Princeton: Princeton University Press. 1948.
12. Sheffer M.S. Presidential war powers and the war on terrorism: are we destined to repeat our mistakes? *White House Studies*, Fall 2003.
13. Dean J.W. Presidential powers in times of emergency: could terrorism result in a constitutional dictator? (accessed via www.findlaw.com). 2002.
14. Schlesinger A.M. Jr. *War and the American presidency.* London: W.W. Norton. 2004.
15. Bush G.W. To the Congress of the United States. Office of the Press Secretary, The White House. 14 September 2001(a) (accessed via www.whitehouse.gov).
16. Woodward B. *Bush at war.* London: Pocket Books. 2003.
17. Bush G.W. The President's State of the Union Address. Office of the Press Secretary, White House. 29 January 2002 (accessed via www.whitehouse.gov).
18. The Government of the United States. *The National Security Strategy of the United States 2002.* September 2002.
19. Schmitt G., Donnelly T. Memorandum to Opinion Leaders. Project for the New American Century. 30 January 2002.
20. Evans G., Newham J. *The Penguin Dictionary of International Relations.* London: Penguin Books. 1998.
21. Pipes D. *Militant Islam Reaches America.* New York: W.W. Norton. 2002.
22. Hurrell A. There are no rules – international order after September 11th. *International Relations* **16** (2): 185–204. 2002.
23. Guzzini S. Foreign Policy without diplomacy: The Bush Administration at a crossroads. *International Relations* **16** (2): 291–297. 2002.
24. US Department of State-Office of the Coordinator for Counterterrorism. Country Reports on Terrorism 2004. Washington DC. April 2005.
25. Gaddis J.L. Grand Strategy in the Second Term. Foreign Affairs, pp.2–15. 2005.

26. Light M. The Response to 11.9 and the lessons of history. *International Relations* **16** (2): 275–280. 2002.

27. Geyer R. European integration, complexity and the revision of theory. *Journal of Common Market Studies* **41** (1): 15–35. 2003.

28. Rihani S. Exploding the myths of terrorism. On: Global Complexity. 2002. Accessed via globalcomplexity.org/terrorism.htm. Accessed 1 September 2005.

29. Burke J. *Al-Qaeda – The True Story of radical Islam*. London: Penguin Books. 2004.

30. Rihani S. Hate of the USA? On: Global Complexity. 2003. Accessed via globalcomplexity.org. Accessed 1 September 2005.

31. Gaddis J.L. On leadership and listening. *Hoover Digest Online* No. 4: Fall 2001. Stanford University: Hoover Institution.

32. Blair, T. Speech in the House of Commons opening the Iraq debate on 18 March 2003. Accessed via http://www.number-10.gov.uk/output/Page3109.asp.

33. Bush G.W. President Discusses War on Terror at FBI Academy. Office of the Press Secretary, The White House. 11 July 2005. Accessed via www.whitehouse.gov.

34. UNDP. *Human Development Report 1998. Consumption for human development*. Oxford: Oxford University Press. 1998.

35. UNDP. *Human Development Report 2005. International cooperation at a crossroads: Aid, trade and security in an unequal world*. Oxford: Oxford University Press. 2005.

36. Coveney P., Highfield R. *Frontiers of Complexity: The search for order in a chaotic world*. London: Faber & Faber. 1996.

37. Byrne D. *Complexity Theory and the Social Sciences – An Introduction*. London: Routledge. 1998.

38. Gilpin R. *The Political Economy of International Relations*. New Jersey: Princetown University Press. 1987.

39. Wallerstein I. The rise and future demise of the world capitalist system: concepts for a comparative analysis. In: *From Modernization to Globalisation: Reader* (eds J.T. Roberts and A. Hite), pp.190–210. Oxford: Blackwell. 2000.

40. Rostow W. The stages of economic growth: a non-communist manifesto. In: *From Modernization to Globalisation: Reader* (eds J.T. Roberts and A. Hite), pp.100–110. Oxford: Blackwell. 2000.

41. McMichael P. Globalization: Myths and realities. *From Modernization to Globalisation: Reader* (eds J.T. Roberts and A. Hite), pp.274–291. Oxford: Blackwell. 2000.

42. Thomas C. Poverty, development and hunger. In: *The Globalization of World Politics*, 2nd edition (eds J. Baylis and J.S. Smith), pp.559–581. Oxford: Oxford University Press. 2001.

43. Murakami Y. *An Anticlassical Political-Economic Analysis* (trans. Yamamura K.). California: Stanford University Press. 1996.

44. Lorenz E. *The Essence of Chaos*. Seattle: University of Washington Press. 1993.

45. Rihani S., Geyer R. Complexity: an appropriate framework for development? *Progress in Development Studies* **1** (3): 237–245. 2001.

46. Rihani S. Complexity theory: a new framework for development is in the offing. *Progress in Development Studies* **5** (1): 54–61. 2005.

47. Gaddis J.L. *The Landscape of History*. Oxford: Oxford University Press. 2002.

48. Rihani S. Implications of adopting a complexity framework for development. *Progress in Development Studies* **2** (2): 133–143. 2002.

49. Harrison, L. *Under-development is a State of Mind: The Latin American case*. Harvard: Harvard University Press. 1985.

CHAPTER 7

Multi-agent systems and complexity

Edited by Peter McBurney

Introduction

In its brief history, computer science has enjoyed several different metaphors for the notion of *computation*. From the time of Charles Babbage in the 19th century until the mid-1960s, most people thought of computation as *calculation*, or operations undertaken on numbers. With widespread digital storage and manipulation of non-numerical information from the 1960s onwards, computation was re-conceptualised more generally as *information processing* or operations not only on numbers, but also on text, sound and image data. This metaphor for computation is probably still the prevailing view among people who are not computer scientists. From the late 1970s, with the development of various forms of machine intelligence a yet more general metaphor of computation as *cognition* became widespread, at least among computer scientists. The fruits of this metaphor have been realised, for example, in the advanced artificial intelligence technologies that have now been a standard part of desktop computer operating systems, such as Microsoft Windows, since the mid-1990s. Intelligent, decision-making computer systems are now deployed across modern economies, from automated stock-trading systems to aircraft landing systems.

With the rapid growth of the Internet and the World Wide Web since 1992, we have reached a position where a new metaphor for computation is required: computation as *interaction*. In this metaphor, computation is something that happens by and through the communications that computational entities have with one another. Cognition and intelligent behaviour is not something that a computer does on its own, or not merely that, but is something that arises through its interactions with other intelligent computers to which it is connected. *The network is the computer*, in SUN's famous slogan. This viewpoint is a radical reconceptualisation of the notion of computation.

In this new metaphor, computation is an activity that is inherently social, rather than solitary, and that realisation leads to new ways of conceiving, designing, developing and managing computational systems. One example of the influence of this viewpoint is the emerging model of software as a service, for example in *service oriented architectures*. In this model, computer applications are no longer 'compiled together' in order to function on one machine (single user applications), nor distributed applications managed by a single organisation (such as today's Intranet applications), but instead are societies of components in which:

- the software components are viewed as *providing services to one another* rather than being compiled or run as a single programme;
- the software components and their services may be *owned and managed by different organisations*, and thus have access to different information sources, have different objectives, and have conflicting preferences;
- the software components are not necessarily activated by human users, but *may also perform actions in an automated and co-ordinated manner* when certain conditions hold true. These pre-conditions may themselves be distributed across components, thereby requiring prior coordination and agreement with or from other components;
- intelligent, automated software components may even undertake *self-assembly of software and systems*, to enable adaptation or response to changing external or internal circumstances.

Such computer systems resemble those of the natural world and human societies much more than they do the arithmetical calculation programs taught in old-style computer programming classes. Accordingly, ideas and concepts from biology, sociology, economics, political science and statistical physics play an increasingly important role in contemporary computer science.

How should we exploit this new metaphor of computation as a social activity, as interaction between intelligent and independent entities, adapting and co-evolving with one another? The answer, many people believe, lies with agent technologies. An *agent* is a computer program capable of flexible and autonomous action in a dynamic environment, usually an environment containing other agents. In this abstraction, we have encapsulated autonomous and intelligent software entities, called agents, and we have demarcated the society in which they operate, a multi-agent system. Agent-based computing concerns the theoretical and practical working-through of the details of this simple two-level abstraction, and the design, engineering and management of the systems that result.

One impact beyond computer science of this paradigm is the development of increasingly sophisticated individual-based models of real-world phenomena in other disciplines. For example, the development of agent models in economics has enabled the emergence of a new branch of the discipline called agent-based computational economics, which has enabled simulation testing of new auction designs, of hypotheses about human economic behaviour, and of economic models of particular market places. In particular, agent-based computational economics has supported the study of markets and economies as complex adaptive systems (see, for example, [1]), rather than as hydraulistic machines with deterministic relationships between flows. Similarly, agent-based or individual-based computational models are increasingly common in biology and ecology [2].

This section presents a snapshot of the topics now explored by computer scientists and researchers in application domains using multi-agent approaches. The five sections here arose from papers presented at the workshop on Multi-Agent Systems and Complexity:

- Jean-Pierre Georgé, Marie-Pierre Gleizes and Pierre Glize discuss co-operative self-organising mechanisms;
- Carlos Gershenson discusses methodologies for designing and engineering self-organising systems;

- Jeffrey Johnson and Pejman Iravani consider complexity in robot football, one of the great motivating problem domains in artificial intelligence;
- Paul Marrow discusses the influence of ideas from biology in the design of software agents; and
- Gilberto Tadeu Lima and Gustavo Gomes de Freitas explore the macrodynamics of financial stability and fragility through the use of agent-based computer simulations.

Co-operative self-organising mechanisms for designing complex adaptive systems

Jean-Pierre Georgé, Marie-Pierre Gleizes and Pierre Glize

Introduction

Classical software engineering approaches cannot guarantee the functionality of the software, given the complexity of interaction between the increasing and variable number of modules, and the shear number of possibilities. Added to this, the now massive and unavoidable use of network resources and distribution only increases the difficulties of design, stability and maintenance. This state is of interest to an increasing number of industrials and academics, including IBM who wrote in a much-relayed manifesto: '*Even if we could somehow come up with enough skilled people, the complexity is growing beyond human ability to manage it. [...] Pinpointing root causes of failures becomes more difficult, while finding ways of increasing system efficiency generates problems with more variables than any human can hope to solve. Without new approaches, things will only get worse*' [3]. These types of application are what we call *neo-computing problems*, namely: autonomic computing, pervasive computing, ubiquitous computing, emergent computation, ambient intelligence, amorphous computing ... . This set of problems has in common the inability to define the global function to achieve, and by consequence to specify at the design phase a derived evaluation function for the learning process. These *neo-computing systems* are characterised by :

- a great number of interacting components (intelligent objects, agents, software);
- a variable number of these components during runtime (open system);
- the impossibility to impose a global control;
- an evolving and unpredictable environment;
- a functional adequate behaviour in the environment.

Our interests

To answer these requirements, we choose to explore the engineering of systems having adequate emergent functionalities. This approach leads us to:

- define what is an emergent phenomena for artificial software systems;
- explore self-organising mechanisms enabling adequate emergence;
- ponder on how to design the decision process of an agent in order to:
  - enable the agent to take decisions with only local perceptions and knowledge;
  - guarantee a coherent and adequate behaviour at the global level (system level);
  - guarantee the autonomy at the agent level (really decentralised systems);

■ define means to observe the designed systems and evaluate their properties (adequacy, convergence, homoeostasis, robustness, adaptivity…).

Our team, called SMAC (Co-operative Multi-Agent Systems, www.irit.fr/SMAC), has essentially been working on the adaptive multi-agent systems (AMAS) theory since 1987. The main topics of interest are the design of complex systems with emergent functionality. Usually, classical design of computational systems requires some important initial knowledge: first, the exact purpose of the system; and second, every interaction to which the system may be confronted in the future. On the contrary, our research concerns theories and methods based on a multi-agent approach in which the global function emerges from the evolving reorganisation between the agents [4–6].

The AMAS theory

As long as the system is not functionally adequate (i.e. does not show the right behaviour), some conditions necessarily occur that will lead to its reorganisation. From an observer's viewpoint, the whole system is able to detect any non-co-operative state coming from the occurrence of novelty or resulting from a feedback returned by the environment concerning a previously erroneous response of the system. Designing a co-operative multi-agent system consists of defining for each component – the agents – all the possible non-co-operative states and the associated actions to suppress them. When the system is running in a dynamic environment, an internal process consisting of modifying the relations between agents is observed. Thus, the reorganisation between the partial functions realised by each agent leads to a modification of the global system function, and non-co-operative states due to unexpected events are progressively suppressed. In this approach, the goal of each autonomous agent is to find the right place within the organisation in order to co-operatively interact with others. The autonomous agent behaviour results from the skills, aptitudes, representations (beliefs) and social attitude (led by co-operation) it possesses at a certain time.

The designer provides the agents with local criteria to discern between co-operative and non-co-operative situations. The detection and then elimination of NCS between agents constitute the engine of self-organisation. Depending on the real-time interactions the MAS has with its environment, the organisation emerges between its agents and constitutes an answer to the aforementioned difficulties (cf. Introduction); indeed, there is no global control of the system. In itself, the emergent organisation is an observable organisation that has not been given first by the designer of the system. Each agent computes a partial function f_{p_i}, but the combination of all the partial functions produces the global emergent function f_S (cf. Figure 7.1). In principle, the emerging purpose of a system is not recognisable by the system itself; its only criterion must be of strictly local nature (relative to the activity of the parts that make it up). By respecting this, the *AMAS* theory aims at being a theory of emergence.

The *AMAS* theory is currently used to solve complex problems in the following domains:

■ Computational biology: molecule folding, ontogenesis and plasticity of a neural network, functional organisation of genes in micro-organisms. The *AMAS* theory allows to define a full creation process of a neural network able to realise a global function from an initial empty system [7].

- Management: time tabling, supply chaining. These optimisation problems with constraints can be solved by a co-operative process between agents representing variables of the domain [8].
- Aided design: autonomous design of aeronautical mechanisms, preliminary aircraft design, emergent programming. For example, mechanical components must find autonomously a relevant organisation to achieve a given global function from a process of a local self-assembly [9].
- Adaptive profiling and information research. In this field, agents representing end-users or providers must learn in real time relevant beliefs on others to usefully interact collectively [10].

Conclusion

The *AMAS* theory is a guide to design adaptive collectives in a simplified manner because designing is of a constructive nature. Instead of starting from the global collective function and decomposing it into more elementary functions, we start by designing agents (their elementary functions) as well as the local criteria and behaviours that will guide their collective reorganisation. This is the detection and treatment of non-co-operative situations. This theory strongly relies on emergence: the agents learn in a collective and non-predefined way. They modify their organisation in relation to disturbing interactions with the environment and thus their global function. Quite a few other applications showed the adequacy of this emergent approach for managing adaptation and complexity in artificial systems, but there is still a lot of theoretical work to be done to explore its properties.

Towards a general methodology for designing self-organising systems

Carlos Gershenson

Over the past half a century, much research in different areas has employed self-organising systems to solve complex problems see, (for example, [11–15]). Recently, particular methodologies using the concepts of self-organisation have been proposed in different areas, such as software engineering [16]. However, there is as yet no general framework for constructing self-organising systems. Different vocabularies are used in different areas, and with different goals. In my current work [17], I attempt to develop a general methodology that will be useful for designing and controlling complex systems. The proposed methodology, as with any methodology, does not provide ready-made solutions to problems. Rather, it provides a conceptual framework, a language, to assist the solution of problems. Also, many current problem solutions can be described as proposed. I am not suggesting new solutions, but an alternative way of thinking about them, introducing the expectation of change into the development process to be able to cope with the unexpected beforehand, in problem domains where this is desired.

The term 'self-organisation' has been used in different areas with different meanings [18]. However, the use of the term is subtle, because any dynamical system can be said to be self-organising or not, depending partly on the observer [19, 20]; if we decide to call a 'preferred' state or set of states (i.e. attractor) of a system 'organised', then the dynamics will lead to a self-organisation of the system. It is not necessary to enter into a philosophical debate on the theoretical aspects of self-organisation to work with it, so a practical notion will suffice: a system described as self-organising is one in which elements interact to achieve dynamically a global function or behaviour. This function or behaviour is not imposed by one single or a few elements, nor determined hierarchically. It is achieved autonomously as the elements interact with one another. These interactions produce feedbacks that regulate the system. More precisely, the question can be formulated as follows: when is it useful to describe a system as self-organising? This will be when the system or environment is very dynamic and/or unpredictable. If we want the system to solve a problem, it is useful to describe a complex system as self-organising when the 'solution' is not known beforehand and/or is changing constantly. Then, the solution is dynamically strived for by the elements of the system. In this way, systems can adapt quickly to unforeseen changes as elements interact locally. In theory, a centralised approach could also solve the problem, but in practice such an approach would require too much time to compute the solution and would not be able to keep the pace with the changes in the system and its environment. In engineering, a self-organising system would be one in which elements are designed in order to solve dynamically a problem or perform a function at the system level. Thus, the elements need to divide, but also integrate, the problem.

Elements of a complex system interact with each other. The actions of one element therefore affect other elements, directly or indirectly. These interactions can have negative, neutral or positive effects on the system [21]. Now, intuitively thinking, it may be that the 'smoothening' of local interactions, i.e. the minimisation of 'interferences' or 'friction', will lead to global improvement. But is this always the case? To answer this question, the terminology of multi-agent systems [22, 23] can be used.

Every element, and every system, can be seen as agents with goals and behaviours thriving to reach those goals. The behaviour of agents can affect (positively, negatively, or neutrally) the fulfilment of the goals of other agents, thereby establishing a relation. The satisfaction or fulfilment of the goals of an agent can be represented using a variable σ. Relating this to the higher level, the satisfaction of a system σ_{sys} can be recursively represented as a (nonlinear) function of the satisfaction of the elements conforming it. Now, it is clear that the minimisation of 'interferences' or 'friction' will lead to global improvement. This does not imply maximisation of individual satisfaction (reductionist approach), but 'smoothening' the local interactions. Also, the synergy [24] or 'positive interference' should be promoted to increase the σ_{sys}. The proposed methodology classifies different methods to achieve this, and when they might be more suitable [17].

The proposed methodology consists of five (overlapping) stages: representation, modelling, simulation, application and evaluation. These stages are common in several methodologies. However, a simulation stage is necessary in the design of self-organising systems [25]. This is because global properties and behaviour cannot be predicted from the representation and modelling of the elements of the system. This requires a 'backtracking', where the designer might need to revise a previous stage before finishing a complete cycle.

This methodology is being applied to self-organising traffic lights [26], ambient intelligence protocols [27] and self-organising bureaucracies. The reader is invited to consult a detailed exposition of the methodology [17].

Any system is liable to make mistakes (and will make them in an unpredictable environment). But a good system will learn from its mistakes. This is the basis for adaptation. It is pointless to attempt to build a 'perfect' system, because it is not possible to predict future interactions with its environment. What should be done is to build systems that can adapt to their unexpected future and are robust enough not to be destroyed in the attempt. Self-organisation provides one way to achieve this, but there is still much to be done to harness its full potential.

Hypernetworks of agents in robot football

Jeffrey Johnson and Pejman Iravani

Introduction

Consider two teams in which small-wheeled robots play football with a golf ball. For simplicity, the robots, ball, parts of the pitch, goals and anything else are considered to be agents. The many possible relations between the agents determine a *network* structure: for example, let robot a_1 be R-related to robot a_2 if a_2 is the closest robot to a_1. We write $a_1 R a_2$. In Figure 7.1(a), the robots are represented by *nodes* or *vertices*. Arrows show directed *edges* (or *links*) between R-related robots, represented by ordered pairs $\langle a_1, a_2 \rangle$. The vertices and directed edges form a *network*.

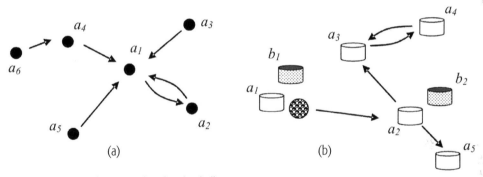

Figure 7.1. Relational structure in robot football.

Networks have many useful properties, e.g. the *in-degree* of a vertex, for a_1 is four, i.e. the number of edges $\langle a_i, a_1 \rangle$ entering a_1 in the network. In Figure 7.1(b), a_i is related to a_j if it can safely pass the ball to a_j. The *path* $a_1–a_2–a_3–a_4$ may allow a_1 to pass the ball to a_4. These paths, if identified by the agents, can be used as communication channels transmitting information among the agents [28].

From networks to hypernetworks

Networks represent structure between *pairs* of agents. However, relationships often involve more than two agents; for example, *defender's dilemma* is that whichever way b_1 moves, a_1 and a_2 can advance the ball (Figure 7.2(a)). This is a relation between *three* robots, take one away and it ceases to be a dilemma. This 3-ary relation is represented by a triangle (Figure 7.2(b)), a natural generalisation of the line representing a 2-ary relation. The notation $\langle a_1, a_2, b_1 \rangle$ represents the triangle,

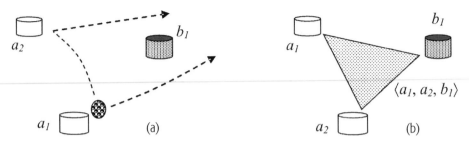

Figure 7.2. The defender's dilemma as a 3-ary relation.

generalising the notation $\langle a_1, a_2 \rangle$. In general, n-ary relations are represented by polyhedra with n vertices: lines ($n=2$), triangles ($n=3$), tetrahedra ($n=4$), ..., (n)-hedra (n vertices) (Figure 7.3). A polyhedron with ($p+1$) vertices is called a p-simplex. A set of simplices form a *hypernetwork*.

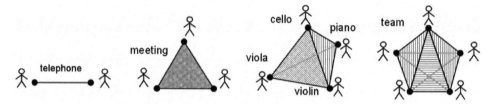

Figure 7.3. Representing n-ary relations by polyhedra.

Skilled chess players focus on creating 'good' positions; for example, in Figure 7.4(a), the 3-ary relation between the knight, rook and king is 'bad' for black and 'good' for white. This configuration is so important that it has its own name, the *knight fork*.

The 'knight fork' relation maps the *set* of pieces at one level to a *structured set* (polyhedron) at a higher level (Figure 7.4(b)). In general, n-ary relations map elements at one level of representation to *named* structures at a higher level. The named structures may be treated as elements at the higher level.

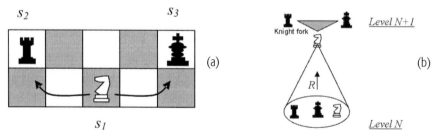

Figure 7.4. The *knight-fork* relation in chess is so good that it has its own name.

The *position* of a robot can be on the pixel grid of the sensing camera, or larger areas such as squares just big enough for a robot to fit inside (Figure 7.5). The relation between the robots and the squares is similar to that between the pieces and the squares in chess. Here, the position is 'good' for the grey team but 'bad' for the black team. This structure (Figure 7.5(a)) can be recognised as important, as it may easily lead to scoring positions (Figure 7.5(b)). Law and Johnson [29] proposed a *space-possession game* in which players move themselves to occupy the maximum possible area.

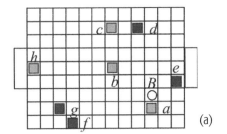 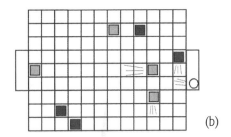

(a)   (b)

Figure 7.5. Robot football is analogous to a dynamic form of chess.

Connectivity: stars, hubs and maximal rectangles

In networks, connectivity is very important, allowing changes to be transmitted between nodes. Hypernetworks have *multidimensional connectivity* (Figure 7.6). The tetrahedron s_1 shares a 1-dimensional face (edge) with triangle s_2, which shares a 1-dimensional face with tetrahedron s_3, which shares a 1-dimensional face with triangle s_4. Thus s_1, s_2, s_3 and s_4 ere defined to be *1-connected*. The tetrahedra s_6 and s_7 share a 2-dimensional face (triangle) and are *2-connected*. Both share a 1-dimensional face with s_5, and s_5, s_6 and s_7 are 1-connected. Since s_4 and s_5 share a 0-dimensional face (vertex), they are defined to be 0-connected. Thus all the polyhedra are 0-connected.

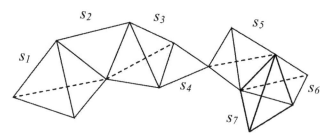

Figure 7.6. Polyhedra connected through their shared faces.

This connectivity is based on *pairs* of simplices. More generally, the intersection of *sets* of simplices leads to the concept of stars and hubs; for example, the simplices $\langle a, b, c, d \rangle$, $\langle a, b, c, e \rangle$, $\langle a, b, c, f \rangle$ and $\langle a, b, c, g \rangle$ (Figure 7.7(b)) share the face $\langle a, b, c \rangle$. The set of the four simplices is called a *star* and their intersection is called their *hub* (Figure 7.7(a)).

Figure 7.8(b) shows 39 shapes in Escher's *Sky and Water* (Figure 7.8(a)). The relation between these and a set of visual features is given by an *incidence matrix* (Table 7.1). Arranging the rows and columns of the incidence matrix appropriately gives the hubs as rectangular blocks of 1s, called *maximal rectangles*.

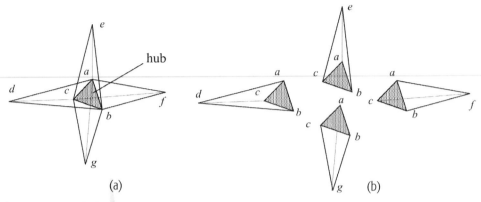

Figure 7.7. A star-hub configuration.

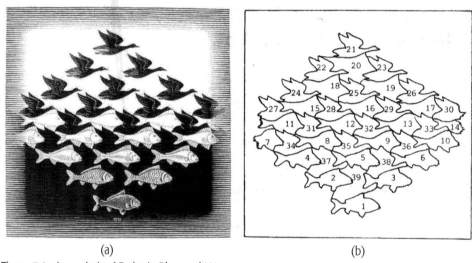

(a)   (b)

Figure 7.8. An analysis of Escher's *Sky and Water*.

TABLE 7.1. The incidence matrix of shape-feature relationships

	1	2	3	4	5	6	8	9	10	11	12	13	7	21	22	23	24	25	26	28	29	31	32	33	27	30	34	35	36	37	38	14	15	16	17	18	19	20	39
scales	1	1	1	1	1	1	0	0	0	0	0	0	0	0	0	0	0	0	0	0	0	0	0	0	0	0	0	0	0	0	0	0	0	0	0	0	0	0	0
mouth	1	1	1	1	1	1	1	1	1	0	0	0	1	0	0	0	0	0	0	0	0	0	0	0	0	0	0	0	0	0	0	0	0	0	0	0	0	0	0
gills	1	1	1	1	1	1	1	1	1	0	0	0	1	0	0	0	0	0	0	0	0	0	0	0	0	0	0	0	0	0	0	0	0	0	0	0	0	0	0
fish-tail	1	1	1	1	1	1	1	1	1	1	1	1	0	0	0	0	0	0	0	0	0	0	0	0	0	0	0	0	0	0	0	1	0	0	0	0	0	0	0
fins	1	1	1	1	1	1	1	1	1	1	1	1	1	0	0	0	0	0	0	0	0	0	0	0	0	0	0	0	0	0	0	0	0	0	0	0	0	0	0
fish-shape	1	1	1	1	1	1	1	1	1	1	1	1	0	0	0	0	0	0	0	0	0	0	0	0	0	0	0	0	0	0	0	1	1	1	1	1	0	0	0
eye	1	1	1	1	1	1	1	1	1	1	1	1	1	1	1	1	1	1	1	1	1	1	1	1	1	1	1	0	0	0	0	0	0	0	0	0	0	0	0
duck-shape	0	0	0	0	0	0	0	0	0	0	0	0	0	1	1	1	1	1	1	1	1	1	1	1	1	0	1	1	1	1	1	0	0	0	0	0	0	0	0
two-wings	0	0	0	0	0	0	0	0	0	0	0	0	0	1	1	1	1	1	1	1	1	1	1	1	1	1	0	0	0	0	0	0	0	0	0	0	0	0	0
feathers	0	0	0	0	0	0	0	0	0	0	0	0	0	1	1	1	1	1	1	1	1	0	0	0	1	1	0	0	0	0	0	0	0	0	0	0	0	0	0
beak	0	0	0	0	0	0	0	0	0	0	0	0	0	1	1	1	1	1	1	1	1	0	0	0	1	0	0	0	0	0	0	0	0	0	0	0	0	0	0
legs	0	0	0	0	0	0	0	0	0	0	0	0	0	1	1	1	1	1	1	1	1	0	0	0	0	0	0	0	0	0	0	0	0	0	0	0	0	0	0

In the matrix the simplices for the shapes numbered 1–6 are all the same, with a block of 1s corresponding to the features {scales, mouth, gills, fish-tail, fins, fish-shape, eye}. All these are good examples of fish. Another group, shapes 1–13, are all related to the hub features {fins, fish-shape, eye}. This includes the less perfect fish shapes 8–13. The following major star-hub pairs can be abstracted:

$$\langle\, 1, 2, 3, 4, 5, 6 \,\rangle \leftrightarrow \langle\, \text{scales, mouth, gills, fish-tail, fins, fish-shape, eye} \,\rangle$$
$$\langle\, 1, 2, 3, 4, 5, 6, 8, 9, 10, 11, 12, 13 \,\rangle \leftrightarrow \langle\, \text{fish-tail, fins, fish-shape, eye} \,\rangle$$
$$\langle\, 21, 22, 23, 24, 25, 26, 28, 29 \,\rangle \leftrightarrow \langle\, \text{eye, duck shape, two wings, feathers, beak, legs} \,\rangle$$
$$\langle\, 21, 22, 23, 24, 25, 26, 28, 29, 31, 32, 33, 27 \,\rangle \leftrightarrow \langle\, \text{eye, duck shape, two wings} \,\rangle$$

The final weak structure is given by the shapes 15–19 which are related only to fish-shape, and 34–38 which are only related to duck-shape. Thus Escher has the fish shapes highly connected at the bottom of the picture and the duck shapes highly connected at the top. Moving towards the centre, the connectivity is still high but less, and it gets relatively low as the shapes lose features and become the background.

Star-hub connectivity in robot football

Consider a robot with n binary sensors. This robot can have various configurations of sensor readings (Table 7.2). In this rather artificial case, the sensor readings give two maximal rectangles, partitioning the configurations so that 1, 2 and 3 are all equivalent, and so are 4, 5 and 6. As shown, some of the configurations have bits set 'incorrectly' owing to noise, but the classification is robust.

TABLE 7.2. A relation between a set of robot configurations and a set of sensors

	s_1	s_2	s_3	s_4	s_5	s_6	s_7	s_8	s_9	s_{10}
configuration-1	1	1	1	1	1	0	0	1	0	1
configuration-2	1	1	1	1	1	0	0	0	0	0
configuration-3	1	1	1	1	1	1	0	0	0	1
configuration-4	0	0	0	1	1	1	1	1	0	0
configuration-5	0	0	1	1	1	1	1	1	0	0
configuration-6	1	0	0	1	1	1	1	1	0	1

Generally, robots are *sensor-poor* compared with the human body. Adding sensors may be an improvement, but can lead to the 'more data – less information' paradox, where the extra sensors are adding no useful information. For example, s_4 and s_5 return only 1, and s_9 returns only 0. These sensors add no extra information, but both add to the 'curse of dimensionality'. More subtly, suppose that some sensors change their values rarely or are very noisy, giving negligible information for the extra computational cost, and possibly degrading the information from the other sensors. Analysis of the star-hub structure can help to detect these aberrant cases, as shown for robot football [30].

Apart from this example, hypernetwork structures can be very useful in representing higher-level tactics and team strategies.

Bio-inspired agents

Paul Marrow

We are living in the future. The science fiction writers of the 1950s envisaged that by the 21st century we would be living in a world full of intelligent technology, in the form of machines performing our every wish [31]. Well, humanoid robots have arrived, but they have very limited capabilities and are not widely used. Meanwhile, the field of artificial intelligence began as an attempt to create human-like intelligence in computers and has developed into an extremely diverse and active field, but has not yet reproduced the full diversity and complexity of human intelligence.

Natural systems show complexity of many forms, from physical through chemical and biological to social and economic; an incomplete hierarchy. Elsewhere in this volume, many areas are considered. Because I am considering how to deal with the complexity of real world problems, I focus on biological systems because they show complexity at many different levels, from molecules through cells, to organs, whole organisms and groups or populations of creatures. Living organisms may appear very simple but actually are very complicated on detailed examination.

Maybe we can draw upon this complexity in building technology to deal with some of the challenging tasks that face us in developing applications that manage complexity. Living organisms seem to behave in a self-organised way, performing complex behaviour despite limited intelligence [32]. Social insects, for example, have attracted a lot of attention because individuals seem very simple and restricted in behaviour, but they are able to combine to produce very complex phenomena such as ant colonies or termite mounds (Figure 7.9). This behaviour has been explained by stigmergy, where individual insect workers follow each other in collective tasks depending on chemicals – pheromones – laid down by workers ahead in the trail. Initially, individuals follow random paths, but when the result is successful identification of a food source, or some other successful behaviour, a chemical – a pheromone – is laid down that attracts other ant workers to follow the same path. The chemical evaporates over time, but not before an organised behaviour can be set up. This is an effective way of combining the activities of many individuals even when their individual behaviour is not very independent or complicated. Resulting from this behaviour, the social insect colony is a much more flexible and robust structure in a changing environment than a single creature.

Observation of this behaviour in the natural world has led to ideas about how artificial agents can be used to solve problems. Swarm intelligence [13] developed as a field inspired by creatures, like ants and bees, that live in swarms or societies. Swarm intelligence encompasses a series of biologically inspired algorithms where simple agents move in swarms to find the solution to problems. One type of swarm intelligence, ant colony optimisation (ACO), is based directly on ants as its name suggests. Originally used for the design of routing paths in communications networks, it is inspired by ant foraging. It has also been used for many other types of problem-solving such as scheduling. As described under stigmergy above, in a software system artificial ants interact through positive feedback provided by a virtual pheromone which acts as a memory, and negative feedback provided by the evaporation of this virtual pheromone. The combination of these effects results in

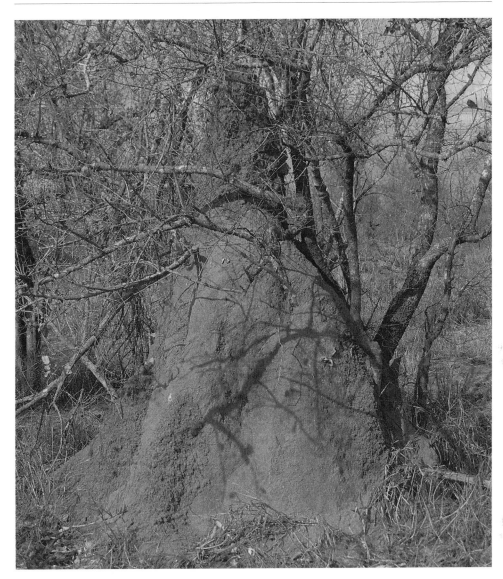

Figure 7.9. Social insects.

selection of appropriate paths by the artificial ants that represent solutions to the problems.

Swarm intelligence uses very simple bio-inspired agents that have limited autonomy. A related but different body of research has focused on what are known as autonomous agents, items of software that can express some independent behaviour (see McBurney, elsewhere in this volume). When many software agents are brought together to make a multi-agent system (MAS) [23], similarities with biological populations consisting of many individuals are immediately visible.

A particular strand of MAS is 'reactive' agents, because most of what they do is react to the environment; but the environment encompasses other agents, and they can react with each other which can lead to the emergence of complexity. When thinking about the usefulness of biological inspiration for problems of complexity, they are probably very relevant because little commitments have to be made about individual agent behaviour.

Simple reactive agents can self-organise in a multi-agent system to produce complex outcomes and applications. An example is the DIET agents system [33]. DIET stands for decentralised information ecosystem technologies:

- *decentralised* because the emphasis is on self-organised interactions between agents rather than centralised control;
- *information* because this is what software agents inevitably manipulate in some form;
- *ecosystem* because interactions between agents were inspired by the networks of interactions between biological agents in natural ecosystems;
- *technologies* because it has been developed as a platform upon which to build technological applications.

The DIET agents system, like the natural world, is built around a hierarchy of elements, from Worlds through Environments, Agents, Connections and Messages that allow interaction between agents. DIET agents have very limited initial capabilities: they can form connections with agents, send and receive messages, and destroy themselves (but not other agents). Although this may sound like too little to achieve complex behaviour, in fact it is the basis for several complex applications that draw upon emergence arising in MASs. Emergence, as referred to elsewhere in this book, is used as a general term for the way in which complex phenomena arise unexpectedly from the interaction of simple parts, in this case software agents.

An example is the self-organising communities (SOCs) application [34]. SOCs, as its name suggests, is an application concerned with helping different users organise themselves into groups reflecting their common interests. But organisation into communities is not done in a centralised or top-down way. Each user has their own user agent, but how can their user agent find other user agents that might represent other users with similar interests? If they can do that, maybe they can exchange information.

SOC uses broker or middle agents which stand in between user agents, but which middle agent a user agent connects to is not fixed. First it connects to one, and sends out a query about the sort of things its user is interested in. If the query can be answered by building a link to another user agent, either connected to the same middle agent, or detected by communication between middle agents, then both user agents get rewards. But this is not certain. If a query is unsuccessful, in that the middle agent cannot find another user with common interests, then the requesting agent gets a penalty. If the user agent that satisfied the query is linked to another middle agent, it moves to connect to the original one, and so the persistence of a user community around that agent is encouraged. As this method is followed over time, we go from a situation where the user agents representing lots of different interests may be all mixed up, to one where they form groups based on the interests of their users around the middle agents. Figure 7.10 gives an indication of this. For more information, see [34].

This is only an example of how the DIET agents system can be used to combine simple bio-inspired agents to make complex applications. The website [33] gives

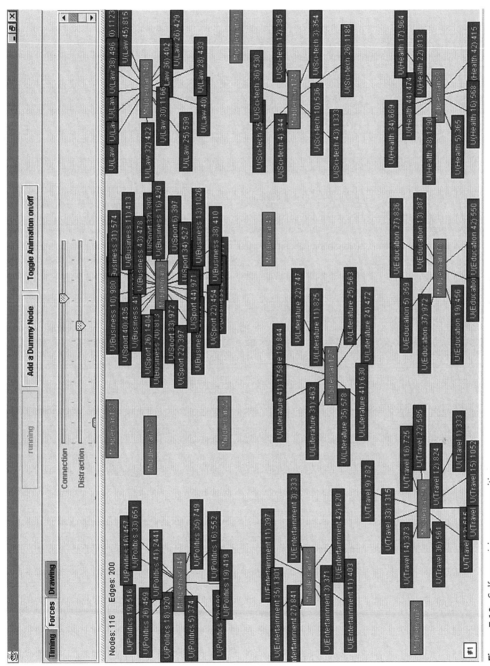

Figure 7.10. Self-organising communities.

more information, and also provides an open source version of the software to those who are interested in working with it.

This section has only had limited space in which to connect the complexity of the natural world with that of bio-inspired agent systems. The diversity and unpredictability of the biological environment means that there are always new possibilities for inspiration in designing agent systems or agent-based algorithms. What is currently a very active research area within the field of complexity science is likely to continue into the foreseeable future.

Systemic financial fragility as emergent property[1]

Gilberto Tadeu Lima and Gustavo Gomes de Freitas

Introduction

We have developed an agent-based bottom-up model, in which the credit supply by an adaptive banking system and the cash flow position of heterogeneous firms are modelled as co-evolutionary phenomena. Systemic financial fragility like that of Hyman Minsky [35] becomes an emergent property, with what we call the *financial fitness landscape* of the system coming out as spontaneous order.

As in a companion paper [36], where a more complete and fuller specified model is developed, financial fragility is analysed from the perspective of the complexity approach, which represents an intellectual effort to analyse the functioning of highly organised but decentralised systems composed of very large numbers of individual components. In the complexity approach [37], these systems are seen as having a potential to configure their component parts in a huge number of ways (they are *complex*), constant change in response to environmental stimulus and their own development (they are *adaptive*), a strong tendency to achieve recognisable, stable patterns in their configuration (they are *self-organising*), and an avoidance of stable, self-reproducing states (they are *non-equilibrium systems*).

The remainder of the chapter is organised as follows. The next section describes the structure of the model economy, and the section after that describes some simulation results. The closing section raises some possibilities for extensions.

Structure of the model

We model an economy populated by heterogeneous firms that produce a single homogeneous and non-perishable good. Firms share a constant-return technology, with homogeneous labour being the only input used in production:

$$X_{it} = L_{it}/a \tag{1}$$

where X_i and L_i are respectively the levels of output and employment of the i-th firm in a given period t, while a is the labour-output ratio. The latter is assumed to remain unchanged, as we abstract from technological change.

1 We are grateful to Caio Racy and especially to Paulo Scarano for comments, though the responsibility for the final content is solely ours. Research funding granted by the Brazilian National Council of Scientific and Technological Development (CNPq) is gratefully acknowledged.

Firms produce according to expected demand, as we abstract from strategic accumulation – and scrapping – of stocks. Because effective demand may happen to be lower than expected, firms may hold unplanned stocks, though. The excess of expected demand over accumulated stocks, if any, will determine individual production flow:

$$X_{it} = X_{it}^D - X_{it}^S \quad \text{if} \quad X_{it}^D > X_{it}^S$$
$$X_{it} = 0 \qquad \text{if} \quad X_{it}^D \le X_{it}^S \tag{2}$$

where X_{it}^D and X_{it}^S are respectively the levels of expected demand and accumulated stocks.

Firms use two sources of funding to cover labour costs – the holding of stocks is assumed to be costless. Labour supply is infinitely elastic at a wage rate, V, that remains unchanged. From equations (1) and (2), the wage bill, W_i, which is due at the beginning of the production period, is given by:

$$W_{it} = VaX_{it} \tag{3}$$

Firms use external, credit funding to cover whatever portion of the wage bill that cannot be covered by the stock of accumulated profits, R_{it}^S, which represents their internal funding. Formally, the amount of external funding, D_{it}, is given by:

$$D_{it} = W_{it} - R_{it}^S \quad \text{if} \quad X_{it}^D > X_{it}^S \quad \text{and} \quad R_{it}^S < W_{it}$$
$$D_{it} = 0 \qquad \text{if} \quad X_{it}^D > X_{it}^S \quad \text{and} \quad R_{it}^S \ge W_{it} \tag{4}$$
$$\qquad \text{or} \quad X_{it}^D \le X_{it}^S$$

The interest rate is set by an adaptive banking system through a satisficing pricing procedure as a markup over the base rate:

$$i_t = (1 + b_t)i^* \tag{5}$$

where $b_t > 0$ is the (risk-adjusted) banking markup and i^* is the base rate, which is exogenously set by the monetary authority.

Firms follow a markup-pricing behaviour according to which their prices are set as a markup over prime costs:

$$P_{it} = (1 + z_{it})(D_{it}^S + D_{it})(1 + i_t)/X_{it}^D \tag{6}$$

where z_{it} is the individual markup, D_{it}^S is the stock of accumulated debt, D_{it} is the demand for credit, equation (4), and X_{it}^D is the level of expected demand. Hence, individual price is set so as to generate a level of expected revenue, $P_{it} X_{it}^D$, which is greater than the total debt service at the end of that period, $(D_{it}^S + D_{it})(1 + i_t)$.

Regarding expected demand, firms follow a set of adaptative rules-of-thumb that differ from each other according to how many past realisations of effective demand are to be taken into account and whether they are more or less optimistic. One optimistic rule will make for an expected demand growth that is equal to the highest effective demand growth in the two past periods. A more optimistic rule will make for an expected growth that is equal to the highest demand growth in the three past periods. Analogously, two pessimistic rules will make for an expected demand growth that is equal to the lowest growth in the two and three past periods, respectively. Two other rules prescribe that expected demand growth should be a moving arithmetic average of the two or three past periods, respectively. Analogously, two other rules prescribe that expected demand growth should be a moving geometric average of the two or three past periods, respectively. Another rule will make for an expected demand growth that is equal to the median of the three past periods. Finally, another rule prescribes that the expected demand growth should be equal to the actual one observed in the previous period. In a follow-up paper of Lima [36], in turn, Freitas *et al.* [38] introduces the following self-reinforcing mechanism. In case a firm remains financially robust during a given number of consecutive periods, with such a number being a control variable in the simulation, it will move to the next more optimistic rule. In case a firm remains financially fragile during a given number of consecutive periods, with such a number being a control variable in the simulation, it will move to the next more pessimistic rule.

Effective aggregate demand, X_t^E, follows a first-order autoregressive process, AR(1):

$$X_t^E = \phi X_{t-1}^E + \varepsilon_t \tag{7}$$

where ε is white noise. The realisation of this shock will be given by a component, X_t^E, multiplied by a value μ_t, drawn from a zero mean normal distribution, with $\mu_t \in (-3,3)$. In each period, the realisation of effective aggregate demand is distributed uniformly among consumers. Each one of these consumers will make phone calls to firms so as to learn about the price. Having made all these phone calls, consumers will call back to the firm whose price is the lowest. In case the lowest-price firm is unable to satisfy all of the effective demand submitted by a consumer, she will call back the second lowest-price firm – and so on, if necessary – to complete her purchase.

Firm-specific markups are given in any period, but they will change over periods according to the following mechanism of local inference. In the end of the period, a fraction of the firms that ranked highest for accumulated debt will then make phone calls to four competitors – pretending to be consumers, let us say – to learn about the price they had charged. Each one of these firms will compare the average current price of these competitors with its own. In case its own price is higher (lower) than such an average price, the firm will lower (raise) its markup for the next period by 10%.

The banking markup is given in any period but will change over periods according to an indicator of non-performing loans, while the base rate remains constant. In the end of the period, the banking system will compute a default rate:

$$d_t = (D_i^T - D_i^P) / D_i^T \tag{8}$$

where $D_i^T = (D_i^S + D_i)(1 + i_t)$ is aggregate total debt and D_i^P is the aggregate debt actually paid back. Since the default rate so computed will be the expected one for the next period, the risk-adjusted banking markup is:

$$b_t = \frac{1 + b_{t-1}}{1 - d_{t-1}} - 1 \tag{9}$$

Therefore, credit supply is not subject to any quantity rationing, but only to an intertemporal price rationing. In a follow-up paper of Lima [36], in turn, Freitas *et al.* [38] introduces the following modification. In case a firm remains financially fragile for several consecutive periods, with such a number being a control variable in the simulation, it may not be granted credit in the next period and will actually go bankrupt in case it remains financially fragile for another period. The banking system then takes over any remaining assets of the bankrupted firm, and sells them to existing firms through a public auction.

The end-of-period cash flow position of each firm can be described by employing a version of the taxonomy proposed by Minsky [35]. Hedge financing units are those that can fulfil all of their contractual payment obligations by their cash flows, while speculative units are those that can meet their interest payment commitments on outstanding debts, even as they are unable to repay the principle out of income cash flows. For Ponzi units, the cash flow from operations is not enough to fulfil either the repayment of principal or the interest due on outstanding debts.

Given the structure of the model, this taxonomy can be represented as:

Hedge: $\qquad R_{it}^{S}(1+i_t) + P_{it}x_{it}^{E} \geq (D_{it}^{S} + D_{it})(1+i_t)$ $\qquad\qquad$ (10)

Speculative: $\quad D_{it}^{S} + D_{it} \leq R_{it}^{S}(1+i_t) + P_{it}x_{it}^{E} < (D_{it}^{S} + D_{it})(1+i_t)$ $\qquad$ (11)

Ponzi: $\qquad\ R_{it}^{S}(1+i_t) + P_{it}x_{it}^{E} < D_{it}^{S} + D_{it}$ $\qquad\qquad\qquad$ (12)

Simulation results

We simulate a setting with one bank, 100 firms and 5,000 consumers over 500 periods. The base rate is set at 1%. The initial realisation of effective aggregate demand is equal to 200,000, with a trend given by $\phi = 1.002$, and the initial banking markup is set at 10%. The shock term of effective aggregate demand is equal to 5,000. Individual firms' characteristics such as initial markup, ranging from 1% to 30%, and the rule to be followed to form demand expectations, are randomly distributed among firms.

Figures 7.11–7.13 show simulation results for a case in which the number of phone calls made to firms by consumers, *c*, is 20, 50 and 100, respectively, while all of the

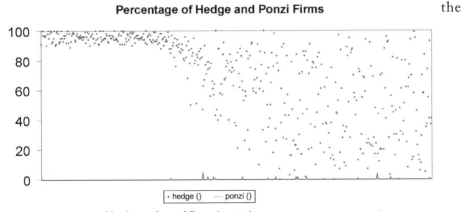

Percentage of Hedge and Ponzi Firms

Figure 7.11. Percentage of hedge and ponsi firms (*c* = 20).

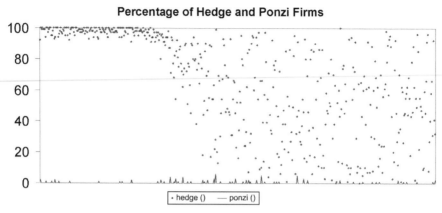

Figure 7.12. Percentage of hedge and ponsi firms ($c = 50$).

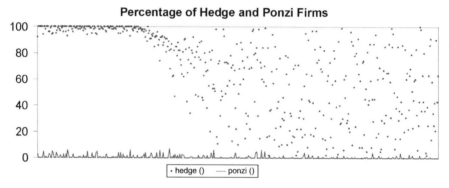

Figure 7.13. Percentage of hedge and ponsi firms ($c = 100$).

firms revise their markup. Indeed, systemic financial fragility becomes an emergent property in a system that remains financially robust for several periods.

Further research

Admittedly, the simplified model developed above can be extended in several directions, and our research-in-progress – for which we invite the reader to stay tuned – has been pursuing all of them. It would be interesting to have an endogenous determination of aggregate effective demand. Besides, introduction of labour market dynamics would allow a discussion of issues related to employment, wage dynamics and consumers' debt, whereas introduction of physical capital as another input would allow the discussion of relevant issues related to investment and capital accumulation. Also, it would be interesting to model the co-evolution of the satisficing procedures of production and pricing by firms and banks through a classifier system and/or a genetic algorithm. For instance, those rules that better fit the purpose of yielding desired results would have a higher probability of being followed; a mechanism of self-reinforcement similar to those underlying Minsky's analysis of the propensity of a market economy to experience endogenous, self-sustaining fluctuations.

References

1. Barnett W.A., Chiarella C., Keen S. *et al.* (editors). *Commerce, Complexity, and Evolution.* Cambridge: Cambridge University Press. 2000.
2. Grimm V., Revilla E., Berger U. *et al.* Pattern-oriented modeling of agent-based complex systems: lessons from ecology. *Science* **310** (5750): 987–991. 2005.
3. Horn P. Autonomic computing – IBM's perspective on the state of information technology. http://www.ibm.com/research/autonomic. 2001.
4. Georgé J.P., Edmonds B., Glize P. Making self-organizing adaptive multi-agent systems work – towards the engineering of emergent multi-agent systems. In: *Methodologies and Software Engineering for Agent Systems* (eds F. Bergenti, M.-P. Gleizes and F. Zambonelli), pp.321–340. New York: Kluwer Academic Publishing. 2004.
5. Gleizes M.P., Camps V., Glize P. A theory of emergent computation based on cooperative self-organization for adaptive artificial systems. In: Fourth European Congress of Systems Science. Valencia. 1999.
6. Capera D., Georgé J.P., Gleizes M.-P. *et al.* The AMAS theory for complex problem solving based on self-organizing cooperative agents. In: The 1st International Workshop on Theory and Practice of Open Computational Systems (TAPOCS) at IEEE 12th International Workshop on Enabling Technologies: Infrastructure for Collaborative enterprises (WETICE). 2003.
7. Mano J.-P., Glize P. Organization properties of open networks of cooperative neuro-agents. In: 13th European Symposium on Artificial Neural Networks (ESANN). 2005.
8. Picard G., Bernon C., Gleizes M.-P. Cooperative agent model within ADELFE framework: an application to a timetabling problem. In: Third Joint Conference on Autonomous Agents and Multi-Agent Systems (AAMAS), USA. 2004.
9. Capera D., Gleizes M.-P., Glize P. Mechanism type synthesis based on self-assembling agents. *Journal of Applied Intelligence Artificial.* Taylor & Francis. 2004; October.
10. Link-Pezet J., Gleizes M.-P., Glize P. FORSIC: a self-organizing training system. In: International ICSC Symposium on Multi-Agents and Mobile Agents in Virtual Organizations and E-Commerce (MAMA). 2000.
11. Ashby W.R. *An Introduction to Cybernetics.* London: Chapman & Hall. 1956.
12. Beer S. *Decision and Control.* New York: John Wiley. 1966.
13. Bonabeau E., Dorigo M., Theraulaz G. *Swarm Intelligence: From natural to artificial systems.* New York: Oxford University Press. 1999.
14. Serugendo Di Marzo G., Karageorgos A., Rana O.F. *et al.* (editors). *Engineering Self-Organising Systems, Nature-Inspired Approaches to Software Engineering.* Springer. 2004. 2977 of Lecture Notes in Computer Science.
15. Zambonelli F., Rana O.F. Self-organization in distributed systems engineering: Introduction to the special issue *Systems, Man and Cybernetics*, Part A, *IEEE Transactions* **35** (3): 313–315. 1999.
16. Wooldridge M., Jennings N.R., Kinny D. The Gaia methodology for agent-oriented analysis and design. *Journal of Autonomous Agents and Multi-Agent Systems.* **3** (3): 285–312. 2000.
17. Gershenson C. A general methodology for designing self-organizing systems. Technical Report 2005-05. ECCO. 2006.
18. Heylighen F. The science of self-organization and adaptivity. In: *The Encyclopedia of Life Support Systems.* EOLSS Publishers. 2003.

19. Gershenson C., Heylighen F. When can we call a system selforganizing? In: *Advances in Artificial Life* (eds W. Banzhaf, T. Christaller, P. Dittrich *et al.*), 7th European Conference, ECAL 2003 LNAI 2801, pp.606–614. Springer-Verlag. 2003.

20. Ashby W.R. Principles of the self-organizing system. In: *Principles of Self-Organization* (eds H. Von Foerster and G.W. Zopf Jr), pp.255–278. New York: Pergamon. 1962.

21. Heylighen F., Campbell D.T. Selection of organization at the social level: obstacles and facilitators of metasystem transitions. *World Futures: The Journal of General Evolution* **45**: 181–212. 1995.

22. Wooldridge M., Jennings N.R. Intelligent agents: theory and practice. *The Knowledge Engineering Review* **10** (2): 115–152. 1995.

23. Wooldridge M. *An Introduction to MultiAgent Systems*. Chichester: John Wiley. 2002.

24. Haken H. Synergetics and the problem of selforganization. In: *Self-Organizing Systems: An interdisciplinary approach* (eds G. Roth and H. Schwegler), pp.9–13. Frankfurt: Campus Verlag. 1981.

25. Edmonds B. Using the experimental method to produce reliable selforganised systems. In: *Engineering Self Organising Sytems: Methodologies and applications* (eds S. Brueckner, G. Serugendo-Di Marzo, A. Karageorgos *et al.*), pp.84–99. Springer. 2005. 3464 of Lecture Notes in Artificial Intelligence.

26. Gershenson C. Self-organizing traffic lights. *Complex Systems* **16** (1): 29–53. 2005.

27. Gershenson C., Heylighen F. Protocol requirements for selforganizing artifacts: towards an ambient intelligence. In: Proceedings of International Conference on Complex Systems ICCS2004, Boston, MA, 2004 (ed. Y. Bar-Yam). Also AI-Lab Memo 04-2004.

28. Johnson J.H. Visual communication in swarms of intelligent robot agents. *Artificial Life and Robotics* **5**: 1–9. 2001.

29. Law J., Johnson J.H. The space–time possession game. FIRA World Congress, 26–29 October 2004, Busan, Korea.

30. Iravani, P. Discovering relevant sensor data by Q-analysis. In: Proceedings of the RoboCup 2005: Robot Soccer World Cup IV. Springer. 2006 (In press).

31. Clute J., Nicholls P. (editors). *The Encyclopedia of Science Fiction*. London: Orbit. 1993.

32. Camazine S., Deneubourg J.-L., Franks N.R. *et al. Self-Organization in Biological Systems*. Princeton: Princeton University Press. 2001.

33. DIET Agents website. http://diet-agents.sourceforge.net/Index.html.

34. Wang, F. Self-organising communities formed by middle agents. In: *Proceedings of the First International Conference on Autonomous Agents and Multi-Agent Systems (AAMAS 2002)*, Part 3, pp.1333–1339. New York: ACM Press. 2002.

35. Minsky H. *Can 'It' Happen Again? Essays on Instability and Finance*. New York: M.E. Sharpe. 1982.

36. Lima G.T., Freitas G.G. An emergent macrodynamics of financial fragility and instability in a multi-agent system. Paper presented at the Complexity, Science and Society Conference; 11–14 Sptember 2005, University of Liverpool, Centre for Complexity Research; Liverpool, UK (http://www.liv.ac.uk/ccr).

37. Foley D. *Unholy Trinity: Labor, Capital, and Land in the New Economy*. London: Routledge. 2003.

38. Freitas G.G., Lima G.T. Debt financing and emergent dynamics of a financial fitness landscape. University of São Paulo, Department of Economics; mimeo. 2006.

Further reading

Readers interested in these topics are recommended to explore some of the books and papers cited below:

Boccara N. *Modeling Complex Systems.* New York: Springer. 2004.

Luck M., McBurney P., Shehory O. *et al.* Agent Technology: Computing as Interaction. A Roadmap for Agent Based Computing. Southampton: AgentLink III, the European Co-ordination Action for Agent-Based Computing. 2005.

Zambonelli F., Parunak V.D. Sign of a revolution in computer science and software engineering. In. *Engineering Societies in the Agents' World. Lecture Notes in Artificial Intelligence* (eds P. Petta, R. Tolksdorf and F. Zambonelli), pp.25–77. Springer. 2003.

CHAPTER 8

Philosophy and complexity

Francis Heylighen, Paul Cilliers and Carlos Gershenson

Introduction

Complexity is perhaps the most essential characteristic of our present society. As technological and economic advances make production, transport and communication ever more efficient, we interact with ever more people, organisations, systems and objects. And as this network of interactions grows and spreads around the globe, the different economic, social, technological and ecological systems that we are part of become ever more interdependent. The result is an ever more complex 'system of systems' where a change in any component may affect virtually any other component, and that in a mostly unpredictable manner.

The traditional scientific method, which is based on analysis, isolation and the gathering of *complete* information about a phenomenon, is incapable of dealing with such complex interdependencies. The emerging science of complexity [1–3] offers the promise of an alternative methodology that would be able to tackle such problems. However, such an approach needs solid foundations, i.e. a clear understanding and definition of the underlying concepts and principles [4].

Such a conceptual framework is still sorely lacking. In practice, applications of complexity science use either very specialised, technical formalisms, such as network clustering algorithms, computer simulations and nonlinear differential equations, or rather vaguely defined ideas and metaphors, such as emergence and 'the edge of chaos'. As such, complexity science is little more than an amalgam of methods, models and metaphors from a variety of disciplines rather than an integrated science. Yet, insofar that complexity science can claim a unified focus, it is to be found precisely in its way of thinking, which is intrinsically different from the one of traditional science [5].

A basic function of philosophy is to analyse and criticise the implicit assumptions behind our thinking, whether it is based in science, culture or common sense. As such, philosophy can help us to clarify the principles of thought that characterise complexity science and that distinguish it from its predecessors. Vice versa, complexity theory can help philosophy solve some of its perennial problems, such as the origins of mind, organisation or ethics. Traditionally, philosophy is subdivided into metaphysics and *ontology* – which examines the fundamental categories of reality, *logic* and *epistemology* – which investigates how we can know and reason about that reality, *aesthetics* and *ethics*.

Aesthetics and ethics link into the questions of value and meaning, which are usually considered to be outside the scope of science. This essay will therefore start by focusing on the subjects that are traditionally covered by philosophy of science, i.e. the ontology and epistemology underlying subsequent scientific approaches. We will present these in an approximately historical order, starting with the most 'classical' of approaches, Newtonian science, and then moving via the successive criticisms of this approach in systems science and cybernetics, to the emerging synthesis that is complexity science. We will then summarise the impact these notions have had in social science and especially (postmodern) philosophy, thus coming back to ethics and other issues traditionally ignored by (hard) science.

Newtonian science

Until the early 20th century, classical mechanics, as first formulated by Newton and further developed by Laplace and others, was seen as the foundation for science as a whole. It was expected that the observations made by other sciences would eventually be reduced to the laws of mechanics. Although that never happened, other disciplines, such as biology, psychology or economics, did adopt a general *mechanistic* or *Newtonian* methodology and world-view. This influence was so great that most people with a basic notion of science still implicitly equate 'scientific thinking' with 'Newtonian thinking'. The reason for this pervasive influence is that the mechanistic paradigm is compelling by its simplicity, coherence and apparent completeness. Moreover, it was not only very successful in its scientific applications, but largely in agreement with intuition and common sense. Later theories of mechanics, such as relativity theory and quantum mechanics, while at least as successful in the realm of applications, lacked this simplicity and intuitive appeal, and are still plagued by paradoxes, confusions and multiple interpretations.

The logic behind Newtonian science is easy to formulate, although its implications are subtle. Its best-known principle, which was formulated by the philosopher-scientist Descartes well before Newton, is that of *analysis* or *reductionism*: to understand any complex phenomenon, you need to take it apart, i.e. reduce it to its individual components. If these are still complex, you need to take your analysis one step further and look at their components.

If you continue this subdivision long enough, you will end up with the smallest possible parts, the *atoms* (in the original meaning of 'indivisibles'), or what we would now call 'elementary particles'. Particles can be seen as separate pieces of the same hard, permanent substance that is called matter. Newtonian ontology therefore is *materialistic*: it assumes that all phenomena, whether physical, biological, mental or social, are ultimately constituted of matter.

The only property that fundamentally distinguishes particles is their position in space (which may include dimensions other than the conventional three). Apparently different substances, systems or phenomena are merely different arrangements in space of fundamentally equivalent pieces of matter. Any change, development or evolution is therefore merely a geometrical rearrangement caused by the movement of the components. This movement is governed by deterministic laws of cause and effect. If you know the initial positions and velocities of the particles constituting a system together with the forces acting on those particles (which are themselves determined by the positions of these and other particles), then you can in principle predict the further evolution of the system with complete certainty and accuracy. The trajectory of the system is not only determined towards the future, but towards the past: given its present state, you can in principle reverse the evolution to reconstruct any earlier state it has gone through.

The elements of the Newtonian ontology are matter, the absolute space and time in which that matter moves, and the forces or natural laws that govern movement. No other fundamental categories of being, such as mind, life, organisation or purpose, are acknowledged. They are at most to be seen as epiphenomena, as particular arrangements of particles in space and time.

Newtonian epistemology is based on the reflection-correspondence view of knowledge [6]: our knowledge is merely an (imperfect) reflection of the particular arrangements of matter outside of us. The task of science is to make the mapping or correspondence between the external, material objects and the internal, cognitive elements (concepts or symbols) that represent them as accurate as possible. That can be achieved by simple observation, where information about external phenomena is collected and registered, thus further completing the internal picture that is taking shape. In the limit, this should lead to a perfect, objective representation of the world outside us, which would allow us to accurately predict all phenomena.

All these different assumptions can be summarised by the principle of *distinction conservation* [7]: classical science begins by making as precise as possible distinctions between the different components, properties and states of the system under observation. These distinctions are assumed to be absolute and objective, i.e. the same for all observers. The evolution of the system conserves all these distinctions, as distinct initial states are necessarily mapped onto distinct subsequent states, and vice-versa (this is equivalent to the principle of causality [8]). In particular, distinct entities (particles) remain distinct: there is no way for particles to merge, divide, appear or disappear. In other words, in the Newtonian world view there is no place for novelty or creation [9]: everything that exists now has existed from the beginning of time and will continue to exist, albeit in a somewhat different configuration. Knowledge is nothing more than another such distinction-conserving mapping from object to subject: scientific discovery is not a creative process, it is merely an 'uncovering' of distinctions that were waiting to be observed.

In essence, the philosophy of Newtonian science is one of *simplicity*: the complexity of the world is only apparent; to deal with it you need to analyse phenomena into their simplest components. Once you have done that, their evolution will turn out to be perfectly regular, reversible and predictable, while the knowledge you gained will merely be a reflection of that pre-existing order.

Rationality and modernity

Up to this point, Newtonian logic is perfectly consistent, albeit simplistic in retrospect. But if we moreover want to include human agency, we come to a basic contradiction between our intuitive notion of free will and the principle of determinism. The only way Newtonian reasoning can be extended to encompass the idea that people can act purposefully is by postulating the independent category of *mind*. This reasoning led Descartes to propose the philosophy of *dualism*, which assumes that whereas material objects obey mechanical laws, the mind does not. However, although we can easily conceive the mind as a passive receptacle registering observations in order to develop ever more complete knowledge, we cannot explain how the mind can freely act upon those systems without contradicting the determinism of natural law. This explains why classical science ignores all issues of ethics or values: there simply is no place for purposeful action in the Newtonian world-view.

At best, economic science has managed to avoid the problem by postulating the principle of rational choice, which assumes that an agent will always choose the option that maximises its *utility*. Utility is supposed to be an objective measure of the degree of value, 'happiness' or 'goodness' produced by a state of affairs. Assuming perfect information about the utility of the possible options, the actions of mind then become as determined or predictable as the movements of matter. This allowed social scientists to describe human agency with most of the Newtonian principles intact. Moreover, it led them to a notion of linear progress: the continuous increase in global utility (seen mostly as quantifiable, material welfare) made possible by increases in scientific knowledge. Although such directed change towards the greater good contradicts the Newtonian assumption of reversibility, it maintains the basic assumptions of determinism, materialism and objective knowledge, thus defining what is often called the project of *modernity*.

The assumptions of determinism and of objective, observer-independent knowledge have been challenged soon after classic mechanics reached its apex, by its successor theories within physics: quantum mechanics, relativity theory and nonlinear dynamics (chaos theory). This has produced more than half a century of philosophical debate, resulting in the conclusion that our scientific knowledge of the world is fundamentally *uncertain* [10]. Although the notion of uncertainty or indeterminacy is an essential aspect of the newly emerging world-view centring around complexity [2, 5], it is in itself not complex, and the physical theories that introduced it are still in essence reductionist. We will therefore leave this aspect aside for the time being, and focus on complexity itself.

Systems science

Holism and emergence

The first challenges to reductionism and its denial of creative change appeared in the beginning of the 20th century in the work of process philosophers, such as Bergson, Teilhard, Whitehead, and in particular Smuts [11], who coined the word *holism*, which he defined as the tendency of a whole to be greater than the sum of its parts. This raises the question what precisely it is that the whole has more of.

In present terminology, we would say that a whole has *emergent* properties, i.e. properties that cannot be reduced to the properties of the parts. For example, kitchen salt (NaCl) is edible, forms crystals and has a salty taste. These properties are completely different from the properties of its chemical components: sodium (Na), which is a violently reactive, soft metal; and chlorine (Cl), which is a poisonous gas. Similarly, a musical piece has the properties of rhythm, melody and harmony, which are absent in the individual notes that constitute the piece. A car has the property of being able to drive. Its individual components, such as motor, steering wheel, tyres or frame, lack this property. On the other hand, the car has a weight, which is merely the sum of the weights of its components. Thus, when checking the list of properties of the car you are considering to buy, you may note that 'maximum speed' is an emergent property, while 'weight' is not.

In fact, on closer scrutiny practically all of the properties that matter to us in everyday life, such as beauty, life, status, intelligence ... , turn out to be emergent. Therefore, it is surprising that science has ignored emergence and holism for so long. One reason is that the Newtonian approach was so successful compared with its non-scientific predecessors that it seemed that its strategy of reductionism would sooner or later overcome all remaining obstacles. Another reason is that the alternative, holism or emergentism, seemed to lack any serious scientific foundation, referring more to mystical traditions than to mathematical or experimental methods.

General systems theory

This changed with the formulation of systems theory by Ludwig von Bertalanffy [12]. The biologist von Bertalanffy was well versed in the mathematical models used to describe physical systems, but noted that living systems, unlike their mechanical counterparts studied by Newtonian science, are intrinsically *open*: they have to interact with their environment, absorbing and releasing matter and energy in order to stay alive. One reason Newtonian models were so successful in predicting was because they only considered systems, such as the planetary system, that are essentially closed. Open systems, on the other hand, depend on an environment much larger and more complex than the system itself, so that its effect can never be truly controlled or predicted.

The idea of an open system immediately suggests several fundamental concepts that help us to give holism a more precise foundation. First, each system has an *environment*, from which it is separated by a *boundary*. This boundary gives the system its own *identity*, separating it from other systems. Matter, energy and information are exchanged across that boundary. Incoming streams determine the system's *input*, outgoing streams its *output*. This provides us with a simple way to connect or *couple* different systems: it suffices that the output of one system can be used as input by another system. A group of systems coupled via different input-output relations forms a *network*. If this network functions in a sufficiently coherent manner, we will consider it as a system in its own right, a *supersystem*, which contains the initial systems as its *subsystems*.

From the point of view of the new system, a subsystem or component should be seen not as an independent element, but as a particular type of *relation* mapping input onto output. This transformation or processing can be seen as the function that this subsystem performs within the larger whole. Its internal structure or substance can be considered wholly irrelevant to the way it performs that function. For example, the same information processing function may be performed by neurons in the brain, transistors on a chip, or software modules in a simulation. This is the view of a system as a 'black box' whose content we do not know – and do not need to know. This entails an ontology completely different from the Newtonian one: the building blocks of reality are not material particles, but abstract relations, and the complex organisations that together they form together. In that sense, systems ontology is reminiscent of the relational philosophy of Leibniz, who had a famous debate with Newton about the assumptions behind the mechanistic world view, but who never managed to develop his philosophical alternative into a workable scientific theory.

By making abstraction of the concrete substance of components, systems theory can establish *isomorphisms* between systems of different types, noting that the network of relations that defines them are the same at some abstract level, even though the systems at first sight belong to completely different domains. For example, a society is in several respects similar to a living organism, and a computer to a brain. This allowed von Bertalanffy to call for a *general* systems theory, i.e. a way of investigating systems independently of their specific subject domain. Like Newtonian science, systems science strives towards a unification of all the scientific disciplines – from physics to biology, psychology and sociology – but by investigating the patterns of organisation that are common to different phenomena rather than their common material components.

Every system contains subsystems, while being contained in one or more supersystems. Thus, it forms part of a *hierarchy* which extends upwards towards ever larger wholes, and downwards towards ever smaller parts [13]. For example, a human individual belongs to the supersystem 'society' while having different organs and physiological circuits as its subsystems. Systems theory considers both directions, the downward direction of reduction or analysis, and the upward direction of holism or emergence, as equally important for understanding the true nature of the system. It does not deny the utility of the analytical method, but complements it by adding the integrative method, which considers the system in the broader context of its relations with other systems together with which it forms a supersystem.

Also, the concept of emergent property receives a more solid definition via the ideas of *constraint* and *downward causation*. Systems that through their coupling form a supersystem are constrained: they can no longer act as if they are independent from the others; the supersystem imposes a certain coherence or coordination on its components. This means that not only is the behaviour of the whole determined by the properties of its parts ('upward causation'), but the behaviour of the parts is to some degree constrained by the properties of the whole ('downward causation' [14]). For example, the behaviour of an individual is controlled not only by the neurophysiology of her brain, but by the rules of the society to which she belongs.

Because of the dependencies between components, the properties of these components can no longer vary independently: they have to obey certain relationships. This makes much of the individual properties irrelevant, while shifting the focus to the state of their relationship, which will now define a new type of 'emergent' property. For example, a sodium atom that gets bonded to a chlorine atom, forming a salt molecule, loses its ability to react with other atoms such as oxygen, but acquires the ability to align itself into a crystalline structure with other salt molecules.

Cybernetics and the subjectivity of knowledge

Tight relationships between subsystems turn the whole into a coherent organisation with its own identity and autonomy. Cybernetics, an approach closely associated to systems theory, has shown how this autonomy can be maintained through goal-directed, apparently intelligent action [15, 16]. The principle is simple: certain types of circular coupling between systems can give rise to a negative feedback loop, which suppresses deviations from an equilibrium state. This means that the system will actively compensate perturbations originating in its environment, in order to maintain or reach its 'preferred' state of affairs. The greater the variety of perturbations the system has to cope with, the greater the variety of compensating actions it should be able to perform (Ashby's [15] law of requisite variety), and the greater the knowledge or intelligence the system will need in order to know which action to perform in which circumstances. Research in cybernetics – and later in neural networks, artificial intelligence and cognitive science – has shown how such intelligence can be realised through an adaptive network of relations transforming sensory input into decisions about actions (output). Thus, the systems perspective has done away with the Cartesian split between mind and matter: both are merely particular types of relations.

However, this perspective entails a new view on epistemology. According to cybernetics, knowledge is intrinsically subjective; it is merely an imperfect tool used by an intelligent agent to help it achieve its personal goals [16, 17]. Such an agent not only does not need an objective reflection of reality, it can never achieve one. Indeed, the agent does not have access to any 'external reality': it can merely sense its inputs, note its outputs (actions), and from the correlations between them induce certain rules or regularities that seem to hold within its environment. Different agents, experiencing different inputs and outputs, will in general induce different correlations, and therefore develop a different knowledge of the environment in which they live. There is no objective way to determine whose view is right and whose is wrong, since the agents effectively live in different environments ('Umwelten') – although they may find that some of the regularities they infer appear to be similar.

This insight led to a new movement within the cybernetics and systems tradition that calls itself 'second-order cybernetics' [16, 18]. Its main thesis is that we, as observers, are also cybernetic systems. This means that our knowledge is a subjective construction, not an objective reflection of reality. Therefore, the emphasis has to shift from the apparently objective systems around us to the cognitive and social processes by which we construct our subjective models of those systems. This constitutes a major break with traditional systems theory, which implicitly assumed that there is an objective structure or organisation in the systems we investigate [19]. This departure was reinforced by the concepts of autonomy, autopoiesis [17] and self-organisation, which were introduced to characterise natural, living systems in contrast to artificial, engineered systems. These imply that the structure of a system is not given, but developed by the system itself, as a means to survive and adapt to a complex and changing environment.

The rift became even larger when it became clear that many systems, and in particular social systems, do not have any clear structure, function or organisation, but consist of a tangle of partly competing, partly co-operating, or simply mutually ignoring subsystems. For example, whereas the older generation of systems thinkers (e.g. Parsons [20]) viewed society as a stable, organism-like system, where the different subsystems have clearly defined functions in contributing to the common good, the newer generation of social scientists saw an anarchy of conflicting forces with different coalitions and subcultures emerging and disappearing again. In such systems, there are many relationships which cut across apparently hierarchical layers so that a system that is subordinate to another system, in one respect, appears superordinate in another respect, an ill-defined configuration that is sometimes called 'heterarchy'.

The growing awareness of these two limitations to the systems view – the subjectivity of knowledge and the lack of order in autonomous and especially social systems – promoted the emergence of a new science of complex systems in parallel with a 'Postmodern' philosophy [2].

Complexity science

In the 1980s, a new approach emerged which is usually labelled as *complex adaptive systems* [21] or, more generally, *complexity science* [1]. Although its origins are largely independent from systems science and cybernetics, complexity science offers the promise to extend and integrate their ideas, and thus develop a radical, yet workable, alternative to the Newtonian paradigm. The roots of the complexity movement are diverse, including:

- nonlinear dynamics and statistical mechanics – two offshoots from Newtonian mechanics – which noted that the modelling of more complex systems required new mathematical tools that can deal with randomness and chaos;
- computer science, which allowed the simulation of systems too large or too complex to model mathematically;
- biological evolution, which explains the appearances of complex forms through the intrinsically unpredictable mechanism of blind variation and natural selection;
- the application of these methods to describe social systems in the broad sense such as stock markets, the Internet or insect societies, where there is no predefined order, although there are emergent structures.

Given these scientific backgrounds, most complexity researchers have not yet reflected about the philosophical foundations of their approach, unlike the systems and cybernetics researchers. As such, many still implicitly cling to the Newtonian paradigm, hoping to discover mathematically formulated 'laws of complexity' that would restore some form of absolute order or determinism to the very uncertain world they are trying to understand. However, we believe that once the insights from systems science and postmodern philosophy will have been fully digested, a philosophy of complexity will emerge that is truly novel, and whose outline we can at present only vaguely discern.

What distinguishes complexity science is its focus on phenomena that are characterised neither by order – like those studied in Newtonian mechanics and systems science; nor by disorder – like those investigated by statistical mechanics and postmodern social science. But that are situated somewhere in between, in the zone that is commonly (though perhaps misleadingly) called the *edge of chaos* [22]. Ordered systems, such as a crystal, are characterised by the fact that their components obey strict rules or constraints that specify how each component depends on the others. Disordered systems, such as a gas, consist of components that are independent, acting without any constraint. Order is simple to model, because we can predict everything once we know the initial conditions and the constraints. Disorder too is simple in a sense: while we cannot predict the behaviour of individual components, statistical independence means that we can accurately predict their *average* behaviour, which for large numbers of components is practically equal to their overall behaviour. In a truly complex system, on the other hand, components are to some degree independent, and thus autonomous in their behaviour, while undergoing various direct and indirect interactions. This makes the global behaviour of the system very difficult to predict, although it is not random.

Multi-agent systems

This brings us to the most important conceptual tool introduced by complexity science: the *complex adaptive system*, as defined by Holland [21], which is presently more commonly denoted as a *multi-agent system*. The basic components of a complex adaptive system are called *agents*. They are typically conceived as 'black box' systems, meaning that we know the rules that govern their individual behaviour, but we do not care about their internal structure. The rules they follow can be very simple or relatively complex; they can be deterministic or probabilistic. Intuitively, agents can be conceived as autonomous individuals who try to achieve some personal goal or value ('utility' or 'fitness') by acting upon their environment, which includes other agents. But an agent does not need to exhibit intelligence or any specifically 'mental' quality, since agents can represent systems as diverse as people, ants, cells or molecules. In that respect, complexity science has assimilated the lessons from cybernetics, refusing to draw any a priori boundary between mind and matter.

From evolutionary theory, complexity science has learned that agents typically are ignorant about their wider environment or the long-term effects of their actions: they reach their goals basically by trial-and-error, which is equivalent to *blind variation*, followed by the *natural selection* of the agents, actions or rules for action that best achieve fitness. Another way to describe this short-sightedness is by noting that agents are intrinsically egocentric or *selfish*: they only care about their own goal or fitness, initially ignoring other agents. Only at a later stage may they 'get to know' their neighbours well enough to develop some form of co-operation (e.g. Axelrod [23]). But even when the agents are intelligent and knowledgeable enough to select apparently rational or co-operative actions, they – like us – are intrinsically *uncertain* about the remote effects of their actions.

This limited range of rational anticipation is reflected at the deepest level by the principle of *locality*: agents only interact with (and thus get the chance to 'know') a few other agents that form their local neighbourhood. Yet, in the longer term, these local actions typically have global consequences, affecting the complex system as a whole. Such global effects are by definition unexpected at the agent level, and in that sense *emergent*: they could not have been inferred from the local rules (properties) that determine the agents' behaviour. For us as outside observers, such emergent properties do not necessarily come as a surprise: if the interactions between the agents are sufficiently regular or homogeneous, as in the interactions between molecules in a crystal or a gas, we may be able to predict the resulting global configuration. But in the more general cases, it is impossible to extrapolate from the local to the global level.

This may be better understood through the following observations. First, agents' goals are intrinsically independent, and therefore often in conflict: the action that seems to most directly lead to A's goal may hinder B in achieving its goal, and will therefore be actively resisted by B. This is most obvious in economies and ecosystems, where individuals and organisms are always to some degree competing for resources. Eating a zebra may be an obvious solution to the lion's problem of hunger, but that action will be resisted by the zebra. Increasing the price may be the most obvious way for a producer to increase profit, but that will be resisted by the clients switching to other suppliers. Such inherent conflicts imply that there is no 'global optimum' for the system to settle in, i.e. an equilibrium state that maximally satisfies *all* agents' goals. Instead, agents will *co-evolve*: they constantly adapt to the changes made by other agents, but through this modify the others' environment, thus forcing them to adapt as well (cf. Kauffman [24]). This results in an ongoing process of mutual adaptation, which in biology is elegantly expressed by metaphors such as an 'arms race' or the 'Red Queen principle'.

Second, since actions are local, their effects can only propagate step by step to more remote agents, thus diffusing across the whole network formed by the agents and their relationships of interaction. The same action will in general have multiple effects in different parts of the network at different times. Some of those causal chains will close in on themselves, feeding back into the conditions that started the chain. This makes the system intrinsically *nonlinear*. This means that there is no proportionality between cause and effect. On the one hand, small fluctuations may be amplified to large, global effects by positive feedback or 'autocatalysis'. Such sensitive dependence on initial conditions, which is often referred to as the 'butterfly effect', is one of the hallmarks of deterministic *chaos*, i.e. globally unpredictable changes produced by locally deterministic processes. But complex systems do not need to be deterministic to behave chaotically. On the other hand, feedback can also be negative, so that large perturbations are suppressed, possibly resulting in the stabilisation of a global configuration.

Creative evolution

The combination of these different effects leads to a global evolution that is not only unpredictable, but truly creative, producing emergent organisation and innovative solutions to global and local problems. When we focus on the complex system in itself, we can call the process *self-organisation*: the system spontaneously arranges its components and their interactions into a sustainable, global structure that tries to maximise overall fitness, without need for an external or internal designer or controller [24, 25]. When we focus on the relation between the system and the environment, we may call it *adaptation* [21]: whatever the pressures imposed by the environment, the system will adjust its structure in order to cope with them. Of course, there is no guarantee of success: given the intrinsic sensitivity and unpredictability of the system, failures and catastrophes can (and do) happen, often when we do not expect them. But in the long term, ongoing self-organisation and adaptation appear to be the rule rather than the exception.

As such, the complexity paradigm answers a fundamental philosophical question that was left open by earlier approaches: what is the origin of the order, organisation and apparent intelligence that we see around us [4]? Newtonian and systems science had eluded that question by considering that order is pre-existing. Earlier, pre-scientific philosophies had tackled the question by postulating a supernatural Creator. Darwin's theory of evolution through natural selection had provided a partial answer, which moreover remained restricted to biological systems, and thus is considered unsatisfactory by many. The co-evolution of many, interacting agents, on the other hand, seems able to explain the emergence of organisation in any domain or context: physical, chemical, biological, psychological or social.

Although it is difficult to imagine the limitless ramifications of such a process without the support of complex computer simulations or mathematical models, the basic principle is simple: each agent through trial-and-error tries to achieve a situation that maximises its fitness within the environment. However, because the agent cannot foresee all the consequences, actions will generally collide with the actions of other agents, thus reaping a less than optimal result. This pressures the agent to try out different action patterns, until one is found that reduces the friction with neighbouring agents' activities, and increases their synergy. This creates a small, relatively stable 'community' of mutually adapted agents within the larger collective. Neighbouring agents too will try to adapt to the regime of activity within the community so that the community grows. The larger it becomes, the stronger its influence or 'selective pressure' on the remaining agents, so that eventually the whole collective will be assimilated into the new, organised regime. Whenever the organisation encounters a problem (loss of fitness), whether because of internal tensions or because of perturbations from the outside, a new adaptation process will be triggered in the place where the problem is experienced, propagating as far as necessary to absorb all the negative effects.

In such an organised collective, individual agents or agent communities will typically specialise in a particular activity (e.g. processing a particular type of resource) that complements the activities of the other agents. As such, agents or communities can be seen to fulfil a certain function or role within the global system, acting like functional subsystems. Thus, complex adaptive systems may come to resemble the supersystems studied by systems theory. Such a supersystem can be seen as an agent at a higher level, and the interaction of several such 'superagents' may recursively produce systems at an ever higher hierarchical level [25].

However, the organisation of such a complex system is not frozen, but flexible, and the same agent may now seem to participate in one function, then in another. In some cases, like in multicellular organisms, the functional differentiation appears pretty stable. In others, like in our present society or in the brain, agents regularly switch roles. But the difference is merely one of degree, as all complex systems created through self-organisation and evolution are intrinsically adaptive, since they cannot rely on a fixed plan or blueprint to tell them how they should behave. This makes a naturally evolved organisation, such as the brain, much more *robust* than an organisation that has been consciously designed, such as a computer. The intrinsic uncertainty, which appeared like a weakness, actually turns out to be a strength, because it forces the system to have sufficient reserves or redundancy and to constantly try out new things so as to be prepared for any eventuality.

Complexity and (postmodern) philosophy

Although ideas from complexity theory have had a substantial impact on various disciplines outside the 'hard' sciences from where they originated, in particular in sociology [26, 27] and organisational sciences [28–30], impact on mainstream philosophy has not been as significant as one would expect. This is surprising given that the related domains of cognitive science and evolutionary theory have inspired plenty of philosophical investigations.

One reason may be that the Anglo-Saxon tradition of 'analytic' philosophy, by its very focus on analysing problems into their logical components, is inimical to the holism, uncertainty and subjectivity entailed by complexity. Within the English-speaking academic world, we only know two philosophers who have founded their ontology on the holistic notion of system: Bunge [19], who otherwise remains a believer in objective, logical knowledge, and Bahm [31], who continues the more mystical tradition of process philosophy. The few philosophers, such as Morin [32, 33], Luhmann [34] and Stengers [9, 10], who have directly addressed complexity, including the uncertainty and subjectivity that it entails, all seem to come from the continental tradition.

Another reason may be that much of complexity theory has resulted from developments in mathematics and computational theory. This is not the normal domain of most philosophers. Complexity has therefore been mostly discussed in philosophy of science, mathematics and computation, but not really in philosophy of culture and social philosophy. To the extent that it has, the discussion either ignored a lot of already established work on complexity [35] or made use of ideas derived mainly from chaos theory, something we regard as a very limited subset of complexity studies in general [36]. (Several insightful and stimulating papers, focusing to a large extent on the work of Luhmann, can be found in *Observing Complexity* [37]. The paper by Rasch himself, entitled *Immanent Systems, Transcendental Temptations, and the Limits of Ethics*, is of particular interest.)

A further reason may be that philosophy has somehow always been engaged with complex issues, even if it has not been done in the language used by contemporary complexity theorists. If this is true, the language of complexity could fruitfully inform several philosophical debates and, *vice versa*, ideas from philosophy of language, culture and society could enrich discussions on complexity as such. To an extent, this interaction is taking place in that part of philosophy sometimes characterised as 'postmodern'. (Note that this term should be used with caution. It can refer to a very wide range of positions, sometimes pejoratively and sometimes merely as a verbalism. It will not be used here to refer to flabby or relativist positions, but to several solid philosophical positions critical of foundational forms of modernism.)

The general sensitivity to complexity in philosophy can be traced in an interesting way by looking at positions incorporating a systems perspective. A good starting point would be Hegel. The dialectical process whereby knowledge, and the relationship between knowledge and the world, develops, works, for Hegel, in a systemic way. A new synthesis incorporates the differences of the thesis and the antithesis, but it already poses as a new thesis to be confronted. Thus Hegel's system is a historical entity, something with a procedural nature. The problem is that, for Hegel, this is a converging process, ultimately culminating in what Cornell [38] calls a 'totalising system'. His position thus remains fully within the modernist paradigm.

Several philosophical positions incorporate important insights from Hegel, but resist this idea of convergence. A good example is Adorno's negative dialectics, where the dialectical process drives a *diverging* process [39]. More influential examples, in terms of the complexity debate at least, are the systems theories of Freud [40] and Saussure [41]. In his early *Project for a Scientific Psychology*, Freud develops a model of the brain based on a system of differences that is structurally equivalent to Saussure's model of language. In this understanding, signs in a system do not have meaning on their own, but through the relationships among all the signs in the system. The work of Freud and Saussure, especially in the way it has been transformed and elaborated by thinkers like Derrida and Lacan, has been central to much of postmodern philosophy, as discussed by Cilliers [2: pp.37–47].

Modernism can be characterised, in Lyotard's words [42: p.xxiv], as a search for a single coherent meta-narrative, i.e. to find the language of the world, the one way in which to describe it correctly and completely. This can only be a reductive strategy, something which reduces the complexity and the diversity of the world to a finite number of essential features. If the central argument of postmodernism is a rejection of this dream of modernism, then postmodernism can be characterised in general as a way of thinking which is sensitive to the complexity of the world. Although he does not make use of complexity theory as such, Derrida is sensitive to exactly this argument: 'If things were simple, word would have gotten around', he famously says in the Afterword to *Limited Inc* [43: p.119]. Lyotard's [42] characterisation of different forms of knowledge, and his insistence on what he calls 'paralogy', as opposed to conventional logic, is similarly an acknowledgement of the complexity of the postmodern world ([2: pp.112–140], for a detailed discussion of Lyotard's position from within a complexity perspective). An innate sensitivity to complexity is also central to the work of Deleuze and Guattari [44, 45]. Many of their post-Freudian insights, and especially the idea of the 'rhizome', deny reductive strategies. Their work has also been interpreted specifically from a complexity perspective [46, 47].

As yet, applications of complexity theory to the social sciences have not been very productive. There may be several reasons for this, but it can be argued that many social theorists were introduced to complexity via the work done by 'hard' complexity scientists, perhaps mostly through the work of what one can broadly call the Santa Fe school [1]. Because this work is strongly informed by chaos theory, it contains strong reductive elements, and in that sense it is still very much 'modernist' in flavour. The 'postmodern' approach, especially one informed by recent developments in general complexity theory, could be extremely useful in enriching the discourse on social and cultural complexity. There are, without any doubt, several postmodern positions which are just too flaky to take seriously, but the all too common knee-jerk rejection of anything labelled 'postmodern' – irrespective of whether this label is used correctly or not – will have to be tempered to get this discourse going. Space does not allow a detailed discussion of the different themes that could form part of this discourse, but a few can be mentioned briefly.

The structure of complex systems

The emphasis on ideas from chaos theory has negatively influenced our understanding of the structure of complex systems. Most natural complex systems have a well-defined structure and they are usually quite robust. Despite their nonlinear nature, they are not perpetually balanced on a knife's edge. Theories of meaning derived from a post-structural understanding of language, e.g. deconstruction, could illuminate this debate. For this illumination to take place, it will first have to be acknowledged that deconstruction does not imply that meaning is relative [48].

Boundaries and limits

The relationship between a complex system and its environment or context is in itself a complex problem. When dealing with social systems, it is often unclear where the boundary of a system is. It is often a matter of theoretical choice. Furthermore, the notion 'limit' is often confused with the notion 'boundary', especially where the theory of autopoiesis is used. The problems of 'framing' and the way in which context and system mutually constitute each other could be elaborated on from several postmodern viewpoints [49].

The problem of difference

For the modernist, difference and diversity was always a problem to be solved. For the postmodernist, diversity is not a problem, but the most important resource of a complex system. Important discussions on diversity and difference, including issues in multi-culturalism, globalisation, bio-diversity, sustainability and the nature of social systems in general, could benefit greatly from the work done on difference by Saussure, Derrida, Deleuze and other post-structural thinkers.

The idea of the subject

The Enlightenment idea of a self-contained, atomistic subject is undermined in similar ways by complexity theories and postmodernism. Nevertheless, the idea of the subject cannot be dismissed. Notions of agency and responsibility remain extremely important, but they have to be supplemented with insights from theories of self-organisation and social construction. There are many unresolved problems in this area and some very exciting work could be done here. For a very preliminary attempt, see Cilliers and De Villiers [50].

Complexity and ethics

Moral philosophy has been strongly influenced by the modernist ideal of getting it exactly right. Complexity theory argues that, since we cannot give a complete description of a complex system, we also cannot devise an unchanging and non-provisional set of rules to control the behaviour of that system. Complexity theory (and postmodernism), of course, cannot devise a better ethical system, or at least not a system that will solve the problem. What it can do, however, is to show that when we deal with complexity – and in the social and human domain we always do – we cannot escape the moment of choice, and thus we are *never* free of normative considerations. Whatever we do has ethical implications, yet we cannot call on external principles to resolve our dilemmas in a final way. The fact that some form of ethics is unavoidable seems to be a very important insight from complexity theory. This follows as well from evolutionary-cybernetic reasoning [4, 6], as from the classic multi-agent simulations of the emergence of co-operation [23]. This resonates strongly with post-structural and Derridean ethics [2: pp.136–140 [51]].

Complexity and relativism

If complexity theory ultimately argues for the incompleteness of knowledge, it becomes a target, just like postmodernism, for those accusing it of relativism. This is not a meaningful accusation and has led to many fruitless debates (cf. Sokal's hoax). The dismissal of positions that try to be conscious of their own limitations is often a macho, if not arrogant, move: one which is exactly insensitive to the ethical dimension involved when we deal with complexity. Modest positions do not have to be weak ones [48, 52]. The development of a theoretical position which moves beyond the dichotomy of relativism and foundationalism (two sides of the same coin) is vital (cf. Heylighen [4]).

The intersection between complexity and postmodern philosophy could lead to both exciting and very useful research. One of the rewards of this approach is that it allows insights from both the natural and the social sciences, without one having to trump the other.

Some current trends

The contributions to the session on Philosophy and Complexity at the Complexity, Science, and Society conference (University of Liverpool, 2005), which was organised by one of us (Gershenson), and which we all participated in, provided a sample of current trends in the field. It was clear that concepts from complexity have not gone very deeply into philosophy, but the process is underway, because there are many open questions posed by scientific advances related to complexity, affecting especially epistemology and ethics. For example, research in life sciences demands a revaluation of our concept of 'life', whereas studies in cognitive sciences question our models of 'mind' and 'consciousness'.

The terminology introduced by complexity has already propagated, but not always with the best results. For example, the concept of emergence is still not well understood, a situation fuelled by the ignorant abuse of the term, although it is slowly being demystified.

An important aspect of complex adaptive systems that is currently influencing philosophy is that of evolution. The dynamism introduced by cybernetics and postmodernism has not yet invaded all its possible niches, where remnants of reductionism or dualism remain. Philosophy no longer is satisfied by explaining why something is the way it is, but it needs to address the question of how it got to be that way.

Conclusion

For centuries, the world-view underlying science has been Newtonian. The corresponding philosophy has been variously called reductionism, mechanicism or modernism. Ontologically, it reduces all phenomena to movements of independent, material particles governed by deterministic laws. Epistemologically, it holds the promise of complete, objective and certain knowledge of past and future. However, it ignores or even denies any idea of value, ethics or creative processes, describing the universe as merely a complicated clockwork mechanism.

Over the past century, various scientific developments have challenged this simplistic picture, gradually replacing it by one that is complex at the core. First, Heisenberg's uncertainty principle in quantum mechanics, followed by the notion of chaos in nonlinear dynamics, showed that the world is intrinsically unpredictable. Then, systems theory gave a scientific foundation to the ideas of holism and emergence. Cybernetics, in parallel with postmodern social science, showed that knowledge is intrinsically subjective. Together with the theories of self-organisation and biological evolution, they moreover made us aware that regularity or organisation is not given, but emerges dynamically out of a tangle of conflicting forces and random fluctuations, a process aptly summarised as 'order out of chaos' (Prigogine & Stengers, 1984).

These different approaches are now starting to become integrated under the heading of 'complexity science'. Its central paradigm is the multi-agent system:

a collection of autonomous components whose local interactions give rise to a global order. Agents are intrinsically subjective and uncertain about the consequences of their actions, yet they generally manage to self-organise into an emergent, adaptive system. Thus, uncertainty and subjectivity should no longer be viewed negatively, as the loss of the absolute order of mechanism, but positively, as factors of creativity, adaptation and evolution.

Although several (mostly postmodern) philosophers have expressed similar sentiments, the complexity paradigm still needs to be assimilated by academic philosophy. This may not only help philosophy solve some of its perennial problems, but help complexity scientists become more aware of the foundations and implications of their models.

References

1. Waldrop M.M. *Complexity: The emerging science at the edge of order and chaos.* London: Viking. 1992
2. Cilliers P. *Complexity and Postmodernism – Understanding complex systems.* London: Routledge. 1998.
3. Heylighen F. Publications on complex, evolving systems: a citation-based survey. *Complexity* **2** (5): 31–36. 1997.
4. Heylighen F. Foundations and methodology for an evolutionary world view: a review of the Principia Cybernetica Project. *Foundations of Science* **5**: 457–490. 2000.
5. Gershenson C., Heylighen F. How can we think the complex? In: *Managing the Complex*, volume 1, *Philosophy, Theory and Application* (ed K. Ricjardson), pp.47–62. Institute for the Study of Coherence and Emergence/Information Age Publishing. 2005.
6. Turchin V. Cybernetics and philosophy. In: *The Cybernetics of Complex Systems* (ed F. Geyer), pp.61–74. Salinas, CA: Intersystems. 1990.
7. Heylighen F. Classical and non-classical representations in physics. I. *Cybernetics and Systems* **21**: 423–444. 1990.
8. Heylighen F. Causality as distinction conservation: a theory of predictability, reversibility and time order. *Cybernetics and Systems* **20**: 361–384. 1989.
9. Prigogine I., Stengers I. *Order out of Chaos.* New York: Bantam Books. 1984.
10. Prigogine I., Stengers I. *The End of Certainty: Time, Chaos and the New Laws of Nature.* New York: Free Press. 1997.
11. Smuts J.C. *Holism and Evolution.* London: MacMillan. 1926.
12. von Bertalanffy L. *General System Theory*, revised edition. New York: George Braziller. 1973.
13. de Rosnay J. *The Macroscope: A new world scientific system.* New York: HarperCollins. 1979.
14. Campbell D.T. Downward causation. In: *Hierarchically Organized Biological Systems. Studies in the Philosophy of Biology* (ed F.J. Ayala and T. Dobzhansky). New York: Macmillan. 1974.
15. Ashby W.R. *An Introduction to Cybernetics.* London: Methuen. 1964.
16. Heylighen F., Joslyn C. Cybernetics and second order cybernetics. In: *Encyclopedia of Physical Science and Technology*, 3rd edition, volume 4 (ed R.A. Meyers), pp.155–170. New York: Academic Press. 2001.

17. Maturana H.R., Varela F.J. *The Tree Of Knowledge: The biological roots of understanding*, revised edition. Boston: Shambhala. 1992.
18. von Foerster H. *Cybernetics of Cybernetics* (ed K. Krippendorf). New York: Gordon and Breach. 1979.
19. Bunge M. *Treatise on Basic Philosophy*, volume 4, *Ontology II A World of Systems*. Dordrecht, The Netherlands: D. Reidel. 1979.
20. Parsons T. *The Social System*. London: Routledge. 1991.
21. Holland J.H. *Hidden Order: How adaptation builds complexity*. Reading, MA: Addison-Wesley. 1996.
22. Langton C.G. Computation at the edge of chaos: phase transitions and emergent computation. *Physica D* **42** (1–3): 12–37. 1990.
23. Axelrod R.M. *The Evolution of Cooperation*. New York: Basic Books. 1984.
24. Kauffman S.A. *At Home in the Universe: The Search for Laws of Self-Organization and Complexity*. Oxford: Oxford University Press. 1995.
25. Heylighen F. The science of self-organization and adaptivity. In: *Knowledge Management, Organizational Intelligence and Learning, and Complexity* (ed L.D. Kiel) In: *The Encyclopedia of Life Support Systems* (EOLSS) (Eolss Publishers, Oxford). 2002. (http://www.eolss.net).
26. Urry J. *Global Complexity*. Cambridge: Polity Press. 2003.
27. Byrne D. *Complexity Theory and the Social Sciences – An Introduction*. London: Routledge. 1998.
28. Stacey R., Griffin D., Shaw P. *Complexity and Management: Fad or radical challenge to systems thinking?* London: Routledge. 2000.
29. Stacey R. *Complex Responsive Processes in Organisations: Learning and knowledge creation*. London: Routledge. 2001.
30. Richardson K. (editor). *Managing the Complex*, volume 1, *Philosophy, Theory and Application*. Greenwich: Information Age Publishing. 2005.
31. Bahm A.J. Systems profile: general systems as philosophy. *Systems Research* **4** (3): 203–209. 1987.
32. Morin E. *Method. The nature of nature*. New York: Peter Lang. 1992.
33. Morin E. The concept of system and the paradigm of complexity. In: *Context and Complexity. Cultivating contextual understanding* (ed M. Maruyama), pp.125–136. New York: Springer-Verlag. 1992.
34. Luhmann N. *Social Systems*. Stanford, CA: Stanford University Press. 1995.
35. Rescher N. *Complexity: A philosophical overview*. New Brunswick, NJ: Transactions. 1998.
36. Taylor M.C. *The Moment of Complexity: Emerging network culture*. Chicago: The University of Chicago Press. 2003.
37. Rasch W., Wolfe C. (editors). *Observing Complexity. Systems theory and postmodernity*. Minneapolis: University of Minnesota Press. 2000.
38. Cornell D. *The Philosophy of the Limit*. London: Routledge. 1992.
39. Held D. *Introduction to Critical Theory. Horkheimer to Habermas*. London: Hutchinson. 1980.
40. Freud S. *Project for a Scientific Psychology*, standard edition. 1950 (1895) **1**: 281–397. London: The Hogarth Press.
41. de Saussure F. *Course in General Linguistics*. London: Fontana. 1974.
42. Lyotard J. *The Post-Modern Condition: A report on knowledge*. Minneapolis: University of Minneapolis Press. 1988.

43. Derrida J. *Limited Inc.* Evanston: North-Western University Press. 1988.

44. Deleuze G., Guattari F.A. *Thousand Plateaus* (trans. and ed. Brian Massumi). Minneapolis: University of Minnesota Press. 1987.

45. Guattari F. *Chaosmosis* (trans. Paul Bains and Julian Pefanis). Bloomington: Indiana University Press. 1995.

46. DeLanda M. *Intensive Science and Virtual Philosophy.* New York: Continuum. 2005.

47. Ansell-Pearson K. *Germinal Life: The difference and repetition of Deleuze.* London: Routledge. 1999.

48. Cilliers P. Complexity, deconstruction and relativism. *Theory Culture and Society* **22** (5): 255–267. 2005.

49. Cilliers P. Boundaries, Hierarchies and networks in complex systems. *International Journal of Innovation Management* **5** (2): 135–147. 2001.

50. Cilliers P., De Villiers T. The complex 'I'. In: *The Political subject* (ed W. Wheeler), pp.226–245. London: Lawrence & Wishart. 2000.

51. Cilliers P. Complexity, ethics and justice. *Tijdschrift voor Humanistiek* **5** (19): 19–26. 2004.

52. Norris C. *Against Relativism. Philosophy of science, deconstruction and critical theory.* Oxford: Blackwell Publishers. 1997.

CHAPTER 9

Politics and policy

Edited by Robert Geyer

Introduction

Economics has been called the 'dismal science' because it was always seen as falling short of true scientific criteria. If so, then politics must be the 'miserable science'. With a huge, diverse and constantly changing field to cover, no Nobel Prize to shoot for and struggling to prove that you are relevant, one should spare a thought for the long-suffering political scientist. No wonder many desperately cling to some vision or strategy of order that can explain it all and give them the epistemological and methodological foundations (and respect and fiscal remuneration) of the 'hard' sciences. The main example of this tendency in the English-speaking world is in the hallowed pages of the *American Political Science Review*. Now the size of a small phone book, the journal has the largest circulation of any politics journal and has been dominated for the past two to three decades by a rigid rationalist and linear framework.

With this in mind, it is not difficult to understand why, despite being well established in other fields, complexity did not start spilling over into political science and international relations until the 1990s. Robert Jervis's *System Effects: Complexity in Political and Social Life* [1], L.D. Kiel and E. Elliott's edited book *Chaos Theory in the Social Sciences* [2], David Byrne's *Complexity Theory and the Social Sciences* [3], and Paul Cilliers' *Complexity and Postmodernism* [4], are some of the earliest examples. Since then, it has rapidly expanded but remains a fringe activity to the bulk of political studies. The following sections in this chapter are focused on pushing that fringe just a little further and showing the possibilities that complexity offers.

In the first section, Samir Rihani looks at how a shift to a complexity framework is not only about academic debates, but real struggles between elites whose position is based on a linear formulation of political and economic affairs, and a general public who are continually confronted with complexity in their daily lives but often yearn for the certainty of order. Following this, Adam Wellstead explores the implications for complexity on policy-making and policy process theory. Using the example of Canadian forestry policy, Wellstead contends that complexity helps to capture the multi-faceted nature of the policy-making process and fills the theoretical gaps within the current policy network literature.

Difficult shift to complexity in political economic analysis

Samir Rihani

An enduring but flawed model

People have been sold a fairytale: leave domestic and international political economic issues alone; they pose mysteries that only a few talented individuals can fathom.

This assertion was a significant element in the design principles on which society is structured, a sharp hierarchy with a small elite of 'decision-makers' augmented by a troupe of all-knowing experts at the top. The select few are prepared to shoulder the onerous responsibilities associated with managing the life of the wider community, but in return they must be given substantial powers coupled with high rewards.

At heart, this is what the 'social contract' is all about. Without it, Hobbes (1588–1679) warned his readers, life would be 'solitary, poor, nasty, brutish, and short'. Politicians repeat the same mantra: we will protect you and relieve you of all responsibility; you have little to worry about and much to gain from the set-up.

Advanced societies have added another nicety to the contract. In addition to law and order, economic affairs and then democratic norms were incorporated. With these refinements, Francis Fukuyama declared, the 'end of history' has been reached [5]. Nothing could happen in future that would improve the formula.

Yet another innovation emerged more recently: the line between the political economy and business has all but disappeared. The 'revolving door' allows the fortunate few to oscillate between the two sectors with consummate ease [6]. Democracy gives people the option periodically to shuffle the faces at the top of the tree. Those temporarily out of the 'public sector' could then move into business, while those in business are given a go at public power if they so desired. Dick Cheney, of Halliburton fame and 46th Vice President of the USA, is the ultimate example of this genre, but he is not alone.

A linear view of the political economy

The 'social contract' and the hierarchical structure that it spawned are based on a premise that is now in question following discoveries about complex systems and the parallels they reveal with the way political economic processes unfold.

Advances in the physical sciences, and the extensive scope they offered humankind to control mechanistic systems, led naturally to an attempt to extend the same logic and styles of 'hard' management to social, political and economic phenomena. The product from this particular assembly line was intended to provide effective and timely policies and actions that optimised the utility to humankind.

This view of political economic phenomena fitted in well with the 'social contract' model. 'Hard', mechanistic processes of management were seen as the most appropriate way to control and then direct political economic matters along beneficial paths. High predictability, it was assumed, was possible, and given enough information and expertise, coupled with innate talent, the right results could be guaranteed with reasonable probability. Expressions such as 'drive', 'initiative', 'vision', 'staying the course', 'determination', 'can-do', etc. became sought-after characteristics that distinguished a potentially successful leader from the rest.

But cracks have started to appear in this structure, and the process of disillusionment is gathering momentum because political economic affairs are becoming increasingly more interconnected, and hence interdependent, and less easy to predict and control. The chaos that has afflicted the National Health Service in England for many years provides an excellent illustration of the pitfalls that a simplistic linear viewpoint driven by central control and management by targets could create. Issue areas such as health now exhibit with mounting clarity the telltale signs of complexity. In most respects they behave less as mechanistic, 'hard' systems and more as complex, 'soft' systems. Instead of the 'tame' problems encountered in mechanistic phenomena, one is confronted by a multitude of 'wicked' situations where problems and solutions regularly change and evolve in time and context.

To understand fully the thorny practical issues raised by this apparently obvious technical shift in viewpoint, it is essential first to point out that the 'social contract model' permeates through a wide range of activities, and that it is popular with people at all levels of the hierarchy and not simply the privileged elites.

Ubiquitous model

What started as a 'style of government' affair has now spread to shape received wisdom in many other issue areas, from major and minor corporations to football. The elites in all these fields promote the same illusion. Bill Shankly, legendary manager of Liverpool Football Club from 1959 to 1974, asserted that 'football is more than life and death'. The message is clear: I am your only hope so do not quibble about the cost. England's football manager is paid several million pounds a year for what is essentially a part-time job. His pay is well over 100 times the average wage in Britain. There is little doubt that a good manager could make some difference, but this is well short of the claims they make for themselves.

Rewards to business leaders follow similar lines, and their rewards are increasing at a fast rate at a time when those at the lower rungs of the hierarchy are being exhorted to tighten their belts. Why? By general consensus it would seem they are uniquely positioned to achieve the greatest growth and profits for the shareholders. The largesse does not diminish just because the company is performing badly. The narrative asserts this is the very time when talents able to deal with difficult situations should be recruited and retained at any cost:

> 'A USA Today survey of 100 of the largest public corporations showed a median increase of 25 percent in the total compensation of chief executives to $13.7 million last year ... Another survey of 200 large companies for the New York Times, found the average CEO compensation to be almost $10 million—excluding profits made on stock options—up 12 percent over 2003 ... In 1990 the average large US company paid its CEO about 100 times what its average worker earned. In 2004, that multiple had risen to 431' [7].

Society sees the 'social contract model' as an inevitability

Elites do not have to work hard to maintain the illusion. The rest of society participates positively in the charade that 'born leaders' are endowed with special attributes that allow them to confront, predict, and control what are recognised these days as 'wicked', 'soft', 'nonlinear' or 'complex' situations.

The 'In-My-Time syndrome' (IMT), an idea I first developed for teaching purposes, helps to illustrate the pervasive nature of the model [8]. A person elected or appointed to a top position, anywhere in the hierarchy, assumes that what happened in the past was mostly wrong because the previous occupant had certain failings. He or she then announces the next few years will see some radical changes that will put everything on an even keel. After that the 'leader' could leave in the full knowledge that no further changes will be necessary: a strictly linear view of life.

Life is not so obliging though; it is complex, unpredictable and full of twists and turns. The set-up copes with this by a constant stream of 'reorganisations' and a game of musical chairs between leaders. What happens next: the new leader arrives on the scene and the IMT process starts all over again. The only modification is that the next person will be given extra powers and additional rewards 'to see the job through'.

The public are content with the arrangement because they can sit back and admire the scene, having left the tedious task of navigating life's journey to a competent and farsighted person who is familiar with the terrain. The alternative would be to take a more active part, but they have been assured often enough that they lack the special attributes needed for the task. They feel absolved of the need to get their hands dirty.

An edifice built on questionable foundations

Despite constant reminders to society that the traditional model does not work properly in far too many instances, elites and their flocks are unwilling to probe too deeply into the reasons for these system failures. Hurricane Katrina, of 2005, is one illustration. A 600-page draft report released by a House of Representatives inquiry in February 2006 criticised all layers of government up to and including the President. The report said government action was marked by *'fecklessness, flailing and organisational paralysis'* [9].

According to the report, the entire catastrophe was so easily foreseen – given weather reports and the precarious location and geography of New Orleans – yet the response was so flawed [10].

The above comment by the report authors is significant. It is in line with conventional assumptions that envision all issue areas within a positivist frame: if one gathers enough information then prediction is possible and corrective action is attainable. Weather was known, the strength of the hurricane was known, the height of New Orleans was known, the state of flood defences was known, and the US government had an organisation devoted to the management of disasters. And yet the operation turned into a painful fiasco. Why? In light of actual events, it was obvious that these givens were only the tip of the iceberg of the complexity present in the total system: local versus federal labyrinthine agencies and interests, a presidency consumed by the war on terrorism, a skewed ethnic mix, low levels of income, etc.

In these cases of failure, a report is routinely published that ends with the promise that 'this could not happen again'. Until the next time, that is, in a different issue area, time, and place. The assumptions and design principles on the bases of which most activities are managed are never questioned. With the passage of time they have become invisible.

The topic does not have to be a natural disaster. The National Health Service (NHS) in England provides yet again a good illustration. It has suffered about 20 major reorganisations in 25 years. The steeply hierarchical structure that marks the

NHS remains intact. Names of departments and activities change, new faces come and go, but at heart the basic set-up is unaltered. When asked how one could judge the success or otherwise of the 2006 'radical' upheaval, a commentator suggested that did not matter much as yet another reorganisation will be on the way. This turmoil in healthcare is not restricted to England or Britain[1].

Why did this flawed model endure for so long?

Do movers and shakers realise the premise of the model is flawed? Of course they do, but they admit to the fact only when they have departed the scene permanently. Abraham Lincoln wrote to a friend back in the 1860s: '*I claim not to have controlled events, but confess that events controlled me.*' One hundred years later, Harold Macmillan lamented, '*events, dear by, event*', when asked what was the most difficult feature he encountered during his years in politics. The ultimate futility of the model was demonstrated by Adolf Hitler who announced his 'Third Reich will last a thousand years'. It only managed to survive for 12 inglorious years.

And yet a model that has yielded haphazard results has endured for hundreds of years, and it has hugely distorted the distribution of power and wealth in the bargain.

The elites and their experts maintain that, mediocre as it might be, it is the only model available to humankind. Margaret Thatcher's often repeated TINA (there is no alternative) follows that train of thought. It is an open question as to whether the reluctance to look for alternatives is motivated by genuine beliefs or by concerns about loss of privileges.

The costs of sticking with the present model are considerable, however. The 2003 war in Iraq illustrates this aspect well. The real cost to the USA is likely to be '*between $1 trillion and $2 trillion, up to 10 times more than previously thought, according to a report written by a Nobel prize-winning economist and a Harvard budget expert*' [12]. Analysts have had a go at examining the reasons for the problems that have marked events once the initial successful war had come to an end. None, to my knowledge, have looked at the operation from a systems point of view.

War is essentially a linear process. Given overwhelming force, an expression used first by Churchill when America decided to enter World War II on the side of the allies, the end result is hardly ever in doubt. The various elements involved are reasonably controllable and barring human error the process is finite, smooth and highly predictable. The next stage, so-called peace, could not be more dissimilar. Numerous interacting elements come into play; their motives and modes of behaviour present a kaleidoscope of patterns that are not only difficult to control and predict, but they are also liable to change at short notice. Such systems are now familiar to those working in the field of complexity, but it is an open question as to whether political and military leaders could embrace the same beliefs without a struggle.

Soft management styles for complex systems

Decision-makers are not unaware of complex systems and their disturbing modes of behaviour[2]. However, these systems are anathema to the elites that occupy the top slots in most walks of life. Basically, they strike at the very foundations of the hierarchical edifice that has given those at the top excessive powers and a disproportionate slice of the wealth cake. Their bogus claims of ability to predict and control future events could not be sustained if a shift in viewpoint were to be adopted that treats some processes as complex.

By the same token, it is doubtful whether the average person would find a radical change to the present model attractive. Soft systems of management are predicated when handling complex situations. Even the 'simple' process of defining 'the problem' becomes diffused and uncomfortable. There are many stakeholders involved and they have different visions of 'the problem'. As if that were not enough, in the course of solving the problem the various stakeholders change their perception of the problem and its impact and priority. Problem and solution are dynamic concepts in complex systems, and the public at large have a significant and continuing role to play throughout the process. Furthermore, there is no clear start and finish to the process. The aim is to define a direction of travel and then move forward with regular course corrections and changes of mind. There is no place for the resolute leader here[3].

Fundamentally, managing complex situations is a social activity. The role of leader is important but not dominant. The hierarchy is relatively flat and the chain of command is short. Substantial differences in rates of pay and hold on power could not be justified. It would take a very long time for everyone to adjust to such a revolution.

Significantly, most people find the present hierarchical structure cosy and reassuring. Ideally, they expect their leaders to have the honesty of a saint, the wisdom of Solomon and the courage of John Wayne.

Leaders might not reach these dizzy heights, but then the faces could be rotated at intervals. In the meantime, the bosses could be roundly criticised with impunity guaranteed by democratic conventions. Stumbling along in this fashion seems more preferable to the average person than actual involvement. This is quite a hurdle to cross before a change to soft management systems, appropriate for complex issue areas, could be contemplated.

Do we have to change?

Sadly, the answer is yes. First, the present model is clearly outdated and dysfunctional. It does not deliver results and has not done so for a long time. Second, and more pressing, the political economy is becoming more complex at both domestic and international levels. The feature that the leading world powers most treasure, globalisation, has piled more complexity on complexity that already existed within most phenomena. There are more actors involved, they are heavily interconnected, and the frequency of their interactions is increasing and proceeds at a fantastic pace. Interdependence, and the associated loss in local autonomy, is now the dominant feature. Simplistic end-state models based on command-and-control and targets imposed by remote decision-makers are not only ineffective, but they are often counterproductive.

The frustration experienced by the USA, as the current hegemonic power, in confronting what it sees as the main priorities is understandable. But it is also

3 For a detailed discussion of this management style see [13].

petulant. There is little chance of winning the war on terror through the input of more military power and more domestic restrictions that in some cases infringe traditional civil liberties. The fate of the war on drugs should have been a good indicator of how things will unfold [14].

Clearly, the model has to be radically changed. This will take decades to come to fruition. Governments and leaders could not be relied on to initiate and guide the transformation. There is too little academic work focused on suggesting the outlines of the new model and how the shift could be implemented successfully. Just because it is felt a new model is needed does not mean any change will actually take place.

Filling in the gaps: complexity and policy process theory

Adam Wellstead

Introduction

Within political science, the discipline of policy research considers the practical implementation of decision-making. The discipline has developed increasingly sophisticated policy process frameworks and models that attempt to capture the growing complexity of governance in the 21st century. However, despite the obvious complexity of the policy process, complexity theory has only recently begun to creep into the theoretical debates and empirical research in the field [15]. In this section, following a review of the dominant policy analysis frameworks, policy community/policy network approach and the advocacy coalition framework (ACF), I will explore how complexity theory goes beyond these two theories, reconciles pressing gaps within the current policy-process literature and is a major step forward for policy analyses.

Concepts of the current policy landscape

At present, there are two major policy network 'schools': Anglo-Saxon and German [16]. The Anglo-Saxon school – which has similar tenets in both Britain and the United States – focuses primarily on the interaction between state and societal actors in networks that are conceptualised as an analytical tool for developing different taxonomies of state-societal relationships. By contrast, the German policy network school is centred on the institutionalised, often non-hierarchal, exchanges between the state and civil society actors. The Anglo-Saxon school presents a metaphorical model of policy networks which contrasts with the 'governance' approach of the German school that seeks to empirically examine network relationships. The policy network approach provides a useful way of systematically characterising the structural relationships among a vast array of policy actors, as well as complementing a body of research explaining the dynamics of policy change, namely the ACF.

The ACF addresses one of the key criticisms of the network approach: its weakness as an explanatory model of political behaviour and policy change [17]. Originally introduced by Sabatier [18] and Jenkins-Smith [19], the ACF sets out to explain the process of policy change by considering the role of beliefs and the mobilisation of information in addition to power struggles between competing interests [19]. It argues that policy actor's beliefs serve as perceptual information filters [20]. There are four key elements in the ACF that allow for a systematic comparative analysis of policy systems.

1. Events external to the policy community are considered primary inducements for major policy shifts and constrain the actions of the policy actor.
2. Understanding the impacts of policy change a time perspective of a decade or more.
3. Policy change occurs within what Sabatier and Jenkins-Smith refer to as political subsystems as the unit of analysis, often populated by more than 30 organisations. Within a typical subsystem are typically two to four key competing coalitions within a policy community.
4. Coalitions are differentiated from another by a three-levelled hierarchical belief system. From these belief systems, competing coalitions develop their overall policy direction and promote specific programmes. A policy oriented belief system is arranged according to three distinctive categories: a *deep normative core*, a *policy core*, and the *secondary aspects*. The deep core, which is equated with the personality of an individual, is nearly impossible to change. The policy core belief, which is the basic strategy and overall policy position of a coalition, is possible to change but very difficult. Over a long period (greater than a decade) in which the core beliefs are in dispute, the line-up of allies and opponents tend to stabilise over a decade or so [21]. Actors will show substantial consensus on issues pertaining to the core and less on secondary aspects. Secondary aspects are the instrumental decisions associated with the policy core. A statutory revision is an example of a change in a secondary aspect. Most routine policy changes occur at the secondary aspect because it does not threaten the dominant coalition's core policy belief.

Changing a coalition's core policy belief would eventually alter the basic perception of policy problems, as well as the general policy prescription of an issue [18, 19]. But as long as the dominant advocacy coalition remains in power within the subsystem, belief systems are unlikely to change, and the core attributes of a government programme are unlikely to be significantly revised. According to the ACF, changing core beliefs requires significant perturbation external to the policy community, such as changes in socio-economic conditions, changes in the systemic governing coalition or a change in public opinion. Sabatier and Jenkins-Smith [21] identified policy-oriented learning between actors as another source of policy change within policy communities. Policy learning refers to the '*relatively enduring alternations of thought or behavioural intentions that result from experience and/or new information and that are concerned with the attainment or revision of policy objectives*' [22: p.132]. Such learning can occur within a coalition and among competing coalitions.

Theoretical challenges to policy frameworks

The above frameworks examine the policy process within the confines of a particular sector and were developed with the explicit goal of overcoming a research paralysis associated with tackling the totality of modern governance. The growing scholarly specialisation in such areas as agriculture, education, forestry and transportation reflect both a dilemma and an opportunity. Policy researchers find themselves relying on policy process frameworks, which limited in scope provide a powerful and convincing explanation for policy change. However, there are two significant theoretical gaps: the organisational dynamics and level of policy-making gaps.

The organisational dynamics gap

Policy actors are most often equated with organisations. Nevertheless, only sparse attention has been paid to interactions within policy community organisations themselves. Instead, research tends to be focused on the organisation's role and function in its environment and its influence on determining policy outcomes. Easily measurable indicators such as the numbers of staff, resources available and their skill-sets have been identified as determinants of governmental and social organisational capacity, commitment and competency change at different levels [23]. However, these attributes only represent one component of a policy organisation's capacity that can and will vary. The organisational response by policy actors requires a rigorous consideration of intra-organisational dynamics (e.g. social structure, technology, goals and tasks, environment).

Level of policy-making gap

Policy process framework researchers, who focus on sectors, have turned their attention to those policy actors with direct interests and away from legislative power-oriented decision-making. Thus policy-making analysis is focused on the bureaucratic relationships between the state and a variety of societal actors. This approach is attractive because those in the bureaucracy's middle echelons often influence government direction. 'While not the most powerful participants', Heclo argues that 'these agents of change usually have access to information, ideas, and position outside the normal run of organizational actor' [24: p.235]. However, Coleman [25] points out that by considering only the meso-sectoral level, the macro structural context may be overlooked. Moreover, there has been some commentary concerning the interaction between different decision-making levels [26: p.67]. A contrasting but equally common practice is presenting states or civil societies as holistic; that is, some scholars 'have given the misleading impressions that at key junctures in their histories, states or societies have pulled in single directions' [27: p.98]. At each level, a different configuration of actors and issues is involved that may overlap in terms of organisational membership. If such overlap exists, the capacity, commitment and competency of an organisation will inevitably vary. Moreover, the decisions made at one level may impact on other levels.

The gaps associated with incorporating organisational dynamics and multiple policy-making levels illustrate the linear and reductionist shortcomings of existing policy process models. Policy actors (organisations) take on multiple roles and, depending on their capacity, commitment and competency, may have significantly different abilities to impact on a variety of decision-making levels. Furthermore, policy actors are no longer neatly confined within a set decision-making level, nor do they deal exclusively with one particular issue level at a time. Political power that was previously marginalised moves to the forefront in the policy process research agenda. Thus, policy researchers are confronted with new sources of uncertainty (when causal processes are unclear), complexity (when causal processes are too numerous), or a combination of all three [28].

A complexity-based policy process framework

Policy science has much to gain from the concepts and epistemology derived from complexity theory, in particular the non-reductionistic approach that can

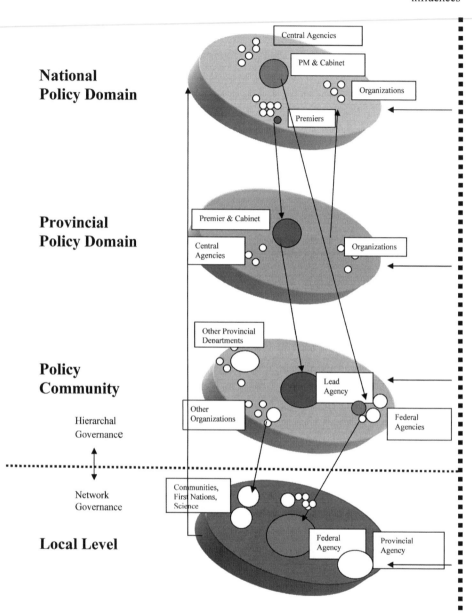

Figure 9.1. Four different policy-making systems.

accommodate a wide range of complexities. Recently, Wellstead [15] examined the challenges to Canadian forest policy within complexity framework. In Figure 9.1, four different policy-making systems are identified: national policy domain, provincial policy domain, policy community and at local level. Forest policy can simultaneously be examined on each level. At the national policy domain level, issues such as trade (e.g. the softwood lumber trade with the USA) are important. At the provincial policy domain, a different set of actors may focus on an issue such as the Mountain Pine Beetle epidemic (such as is the case in British Columbia (BC)), whereas at the policy community level, specific forest management policies may be debated. Whereas Wellstead [15] examined different levels of Canadian forestry decision-making, Figure 9.1 can be applied to nearly all advanced capitalist policy systems. Finally, each individual organisation (policy actor) should be considered as a unique fifth system of its own. The environment (fitness landscape) of the policy community (system) would comprise the other four systems, which remain interconnected but in a less hierarchal and nested fashion. Each policy-making system (level) comprises a host of government and societal organisations.

An early attempt to apply complexity theory in political science can be found in Geyer [29, 30], which used complexity to re-examine European Union integration and the Third Way. His framework is based on a paradigm of order, whereby political phenomena demonstrate a variety of complex attributes ranging from linear to alinear. Geyer's complexity framework introduces the concept of order and the ranges of linearity that characterise general political phenomena. Several necessary amendments are made to this framework, thus allowing policy frameworks to be examined within the context of both complexity theories:

1. The role of causal complexity and additivity. Causality is particularly important when determining policy outcomes resulting from the interaction of phenomena at different decision-making levels. Causal complexity describes a process in which the effect of one variable or characteristic can depend on the presence of other characteristics, or a process in which the outcomes result from several different combinations of conditions [1, 31].

2. In Figure 9.2, the three main components (additivity, different decision-making levels and linearity) that define complex policy-making systems are illustrated. Thus political-policy related phenomena can range from linear to alinear in their attributes. Policy outcomes (dependent variables) occur as the result of the interaction of a host of different independent variables.

3. The role of policy issues is also addressed in this framework. Each particular issue will lead to the identification of issue-specific policy related phenomena as the causal drivers of policy change. Thus, there will be several complexity-based policy frameworks employed that correspond to particular issue areas.

A forest-based policy case study: the Mountain Pine Beetle

A temporal consideration is a necessary feature of a policy-based complexity framework. A massive outbreak of the beetles throughout BC's southern interior resulted in this phenomena becoming an issue extending beyond its forest policy community, but also included the provincial and national policy domains. Furthermore, the phenomena of long-term climate change impacts became better known and thereby demonstrated that the series of consecutive warm winters may have contributed to the beetle's outbreak. The economic well-being of forest-dependent communities became as important to the provincial making domain as halting the epidemic's spread. Also, the provincial domain was impacted by negative public opinion of the widespread beetle damage. Exports and timber supply shifted along the complexity continuum due to the uncertainty caused by the loss of timber ($20 billion timber value), combined with the difficulties resulting from the softwood lumber dispute. In Canada, the importance of executive and interstate federalism cannot be overstated. The BC Premier, Gordon Campbell, directly appealed to the federal government for emergency funding and the establishment of the *Mountain Pine Beetle Action Plan* in late 2001 (British Columbia, 2003). The possibility of policy learning and the development of a mountain pine beeetle policy network emerged in the form of the Minister's Community Advisory Group that consisted of First Nations, the forest industry, academia, logging contractors, environmental groups and the federal government (British Columbia, 2004). The role of science and policy learning can be highlighted by the debate that emerged over the issue of the extent of salvage logging infected areas. Finally, core policy beliefs and policy direction of the dominant industrial-provincial advocacy coalition may be challenged because of an exogenous impact upon BC's forest policy community. This example highlights the variety of political phenomena at play that cannot be accommodated within traditional linear policy frameworks.

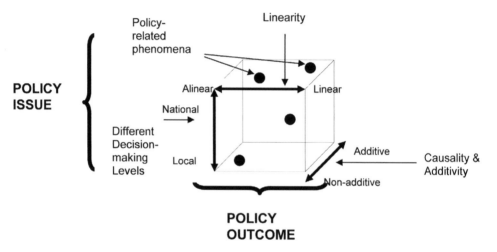

Figure 9.2. Linear–alinear/national–local/additivity continuum.

Implications for policy research and a critical introspective[4]

The complexity-based policy framework introduced in this section is a theoretical response to several serious shortcomings within current policy based research. Complexity theory can help policy scientists to better understand policy change in light of changes to governance in capitalist states. The changing capacity, competency and commitment of organisations in a dynamic multiple level decision-making structure will have a considerable impact on policy research. Organisations will be prevalent at different decision-making levels.

Introducing new theoretical modifications to the policy frameworks that will lead to a considerable 'messiness' was also created in terms of the possible unpacking of

4 I acknowledge the feedback and insights received during the presentation of the ideas developed in this chapter at the Complexity, Science, and Society conference held at the University of Liverpool, Liverpool, UK (11–14 September 2005).

observed empirical aspects within a complexity-based policy process framework. There are potentially many variables and complex causal relationships that could be encountered when undertaking an empirical-based study, particularly a study that seeks to make inferences about political phenomena. An enhanced level of theoretical sophistication must also be balanced and met with levels of corresponding research rigor in empirical undertakings. These requirements are necessary if a comparative research agenda is sought. Several theoretical-empirical bridging challenges will be encountered in future policy research. The first is a locating political phenomena on the linear–alinear/national–local/additivity continuum described in Figure 9.2. A second challenge is fully explaining and justifying the shift of phenomena between different decision-making levels and/or different complexities. Finally, researchers must choose appropriate methods. Geyer *et al.* [32] recommend adopting a variety of methods ranging from statistical to historical narratives. The choice depends upon the complexity of the phenomena under investigation.

Despite these challenges, complexity theory should be able to assist policy researchers in overcoming the above-identified gaps associated with the role of the organisation in a multi-level decision-making environment. The theoretical framework developed here acknowledges these levels, the degree of order that policy related phenomena can be found, and the role of complex causality leads to a variety of policy outcomes. Finally, traditional policy frameworks are not abandoned, but instead are given new life as they continue to play an important role but within the wider context of complexity.

References

1. Jervis R. *System Effects: Complexity in political and social life.* Princeton, NJ: Princeton University Press. 1997.
2. Kiel L.D., Elliot E. (editors). *Chaos Theory in the Social Sciences.* 1997.
3. Byrne D. *Complexity Theory and the Social Sciences – An Introduction.* London: Routledge. 1998.
4. Cilliers P. *Complexity and Postmodernism.* London: Routledge. 1998.
5. Fukuyama F. *The End of History and the Last Man.* Harmondsworth: Penguin. 1993.
6. Hertz N. *The Silent Takeover: Global capitalism and the death of democracy.* London: Heinemann. 2001.
7. *New York Times*, 17 January 2006.
8. See www.globalcomplexity.org for detailed description of the IMT syndrome.
9. www.news.scotsman.com, 13 February 2006. Accessed 6 March 2006.
10. www.nytimes.com, 13 February 2006. Accessed 6 March 2006.
11. Oxman A.D., Sackett D.L., Chalmers I. *et al.* A surrealistic mega-analysis of redisorganisation theories. *Journal of the Royal Society of Medicine* **98**. 2005.
12. *The Guardian.* Iraq war could cost US over $2 trillion. 7 January 2006.
13. Langley G.J., Nolan K.M., Nolan T.W. *et al. The Improvement Guide: A practical approach to enhancing organisational performance.* San Francisco: Jossey Bass Wiley. 1996.
14. Davies N. War on drugs. *The Guardian*, 14 and 15 June 2001.

15. Wellstead A. Addressing natural resource policy complexities and change. Unpublished PhD dissertation, Department of Renewable Resources, University of Alberta, Edmonton, Alberta, Canada. 2006.

16. Börzel T. Organizing Babylon – on the different conceptions of policy networks. *Public Administration* **76** (2): 253–273. 1998.

17. Dowding K. Model or metaphor? A critical review of the policy network approach. *Political Studies* **43**: 136–158. 1995.

18. Sabatier P. An advocacy coalition framework of policy change and the role of policy oriented learning therein. *Policy Sciences* **21**: 129–168. 1988.

19. Jenkins-Smith, H. 1988. Analytical debates and policy learning: analysis and change in the federal bureaucracy. *Policy Sciences* **21**: 169–211. 1988.

20. Schlager E., Blomquist W. A comparison of three emerging theories of the policy process. *Political Research Quarterly* **49**: 631–650. 1996.

21. Sabatier P. Policy change over a decade or more. In: *Policy Change and Learning: An advocacy coalition approach* (ed P. Sabatier and H. Jenkins-Smith), pp.13–40. Boulder: Westview Press. 1993.

22. Sabatier P., Jenkins-Smith H. The advocacy coalition framework: an assessment. In: *Theories of the Policy Process* (ed P. Sabatier), pp.117–166. Boulder: Westview Press. 1999.

23. Lindquist E. Public managers and policy communities: learning to meet new challenges. *Canadian Journal of Public Administration* **35** (2): 127–157. 1992.

24. Heclo H. Issue networks and the executive establishment. In: *The New American Political System* (ed A. King), pp.87–124. Washington DC: American Enterprise Institute. 1979.

25. Coleman W. Policy networks, policy communities, and the problems of governance. *Governance* **5**: 154–180. 1992.

26. Coleman W., Perl A. Internationalized policy environments and policy network analysis. *Political Studies* **47** (4): 691–709. 1999.

27. Migdal J. *State in Society*. Cambridge: Cambridge University Press. 2001.

28. Roe E. Varieties of issue incompleteness and coordination: An example from ecosystem management. *Policy Sciences* **34** (2): 111–133. 2001.

29. Geyer R. Beyond the Third Way: the science of complexity and the politics of choice. *British Journal of Politics and International Relations* **5** (2): 237–257. 2003.

30. Geyer R. European integration, complexity and the revision of theory. *Journal of Common Market Studies* **41** (1): 15–35. 2003.

31. Braumoeller B. Causal complexity and the study of politics. *Political Analysis* **11** (3): 209–233. 2003.

32. Geyer R., Mackintosh A., Lehmann K. *Integrating UK and European Social Policy: The complexity of Europeanisation*. Oxford: Radciffe. 2005.

CHAPTER 10

Social theory and complexity

Edited by Kingsley Dennis and Paul Haynes

Introduction

Social theory is concerned with developing concepts, hypotheses and models with which to understand society, culture and the range of factors that enable interaction between people to occur. Through the course of exploring the socio-cultural terrain, social theorists have made use of a wide range of methods and produced a vast amount of literature examining how people interact with each other in almost every conceivable context.

Although there is some agreement among theorists about individual points of analysis, the one obvious point of agreement between social theorists is that the social world is complicated. Not only is the social world complex, involving the interdependency of many people, and mediated by a seemingly growing number of institutions and ever more sophisticated technology, it is also changing rapidly in identifiable and less identifiable ways. As a consequence of a global sphere that is becoming more globalised, inter-connected, co-dependent, complex, reflexive, networked and dynamic, the social sciences have begun to use other models with which to view these emerging processes. One of these is complexity theory, from the complexity sciences. Complexity theory, which has had a great deal of success in exploring complex interactions in chemistry, biology, ecology, computer simulations and other fields, has likewise become a useful resource with which to enable social theory to explore its own fundamental dynamics.

Concepts that seem on the surface to be related to these complexity themes have a long history in social theory. Indeed some key themes, such as the multifarious interaction of units of analysis, can be traced to the late 19th-century works of Max Weber, whereas other cyclical and dialectical socio-economic processes outlined by Marx can be incorporated into a framework of social self-organisation. It was not, though, until the 1940s and 1950s that the forerunners to complexity were developed into a social theory in a systematic way. The development of general systems theory and cybernetics were quickly applied to 'social systems' (e.g. Bateson; Forrester), while functionalism, developed by Talcott Parsons around this time, attempted to explain the way society worked as a closed yet complex system.

The emergence of complexity in the mainstream began to occur in the 1990s, after the hype of short-lived metaphors, for example catastrophe and chaos theory, and was inspired either by Ilya Prigogine[1] and collaborators, or through researchers associated with the Santa Fe Institute (Kauffman, Arrow, Arthur, Gell-Mann; Holland, etc.), or both. In the mid-1990s a variety of conferences, journal articles and edited collections began to emerge, indicating that a community of social science researchers were using complexity themes, which John Urry describes as 'the complexity turn' within the social sciences [1].

Complexity science, complex adaptive systems or self-organisation enabled metaphors and heuristics to be made, and were themselves metaphors for conceiving of new approaches to understanding social science. The metaphors at this stage were merely suggestive, lacking a clear linkage to pressing social science problems or research agenda, and being unable to outline ideas that problematise unreflective social theory assumptions; i.e. bringing social science, if not into the 21st century, then out of the 17th century[2], on issues such as causality, equilibrium and determinacy.

To consider the complexity sciences entails that we also include an acknowledgement to the presence of the multiple and complex sites where complexity theory is produced and consumed as a viable method and/or metaphor. Thrift [2] follows how complexity theory is itself a metaphorical movement, one that is of a particularly rapid kind. He also refers to it as a 'scientific amalgam', as 'an accretion of ideas, a rhetorical hybrid' [3].

Complexity in the social sciences, and similarly complexity-informed social theory, has itself grown into a more mature research community, supported by the proliferation of specialist journals, research centres, courses and conferences. This was clearly demonstrated in the range and quality of social theory discussed at the Liverpool Complexity, Science and Society Conference in September 2005.

The following three brief articles examine the relationship, validity and usefulness of complexity theory to governance, blogging and social action. In the first – 'The governance of complexity and the complexity of governance, revisited' – Bob Jessop argues that the continuing excess of complexity in the real world is a major cause for the failure of governance. This, he explains, results in the growing interest in forms of governance that can more reflexively integrate notions of complexity.

In 'Complexity and the bloggers: the rise of the blogosphere', Kingsley Dennis attempts to use complexity theory to examine the phenomenon of blogging. He argues that features of complexity help to frame the rise in amateur informational networks, and shows how 'social information-sharing, non-localised formations/ movements are beginning to infringe, influence, and change the behaviours of social practice'.

Lastly, David Byrne, in 'Complexity, cities and social action', looks at the methodology of action-research and asks how to generalise this complex and developing experience to other practical contexts. He argues passionately that contextualising action-research within a complexity framework re-politicises the urban planning process.

To conclude, a complexity informed social theory, coupled with a continued emphasis on the impact of change in the social world, is shifting complexity thinking further into the mainstream of the discipline. This is part of what has been termed *the complexity turn*.

---

1 Prigogine has been also directly engaged with social science in the past decade or so, for example through the Gulbenkian Commission on the Reconstructing of the Social Sciences in 1996 [4].
2 See Kenneth Boulding's remarks quoted in Waldrop [5].

The governance of complexity and the complexity of governance, revisited

Bob Jessop

Complexity is complex. This is reflected, especially in the social sciences, in the status of complexity as a chaotic conception. Thus, I must first reduce the complexity of complexity in order to connect it to governance rather than another topic. Indeed, faced with complexity, such acts of simplification are inevitable for any agent or operating system. This is because ontological complexity enforces selection on natural and social systems alike. One way to classify and interpret such systems is in terms of how they select selections. For social systems this involves simplification through specific meaning systems, forms of representation and limited action repertoires. Thus, we should examine the selectivity of systems and the reflexivity of agents, and explore the dialectic between the complexity of the real world and the manner in which the real world comes to be interpreted as complex. Issues of governance enter here because, if complexity is a feature of the real world (and not just a social construction of particular observers of that world), it has serious implications for attempts to govern complexity. This section revisits arguments about the governance of complexity presented 10 years ago [6] and argues for 'romantic public irony' as a response to recognition of the complexity of governance.

Theorising complexity

Urry suggests that sociology generates hypotheses through metaphor and that we should choose metaphors that best correspond to the real world [7]. Ignoring the apparent contradiction in this position and the risk that metaphors are used to tell 'good stories' rather than provide 'solid arguments', it is a matter of sociological observation that current interest in complexity reflects a *Zeitdiagnostik* that the social world has become more complex. This, in turn, has led to the search for new ways of dealing with complexity. Among the reasons advanced for a dramatic intensification of societal complexity are:

- increased functional differentiation combined with increased interdependence among functional systems;
- increased fuzziness, contestability and de-differentiation of institutional boundaries;
- increased complexity of spatial and scalar relations, and horizons of action, as national economies, national states and national societies cease to be the main axes and reference points in societal organisation;
- increased complexity and interconnectedness of temporalities and temporal horizons, ranging from split-second timing (e.g. computer-driven trading) to an acceleration of the glacial time of social and environmental change;
- multiplication of identities and the imagined communities to which different social forces orient their actions and seek to coordinate them;
- increased importance of knowledge and organised learning; and, because of the above;
- the self-potentiating nature of complexity, whereby complex systems generally operate in ways that create opportunities for additional complexity.

But recognition of growing social complexity, even assuming that this could be measured accurately and compared with other cases than the post-war boom years in advanced capitalist economies, does not justify the simple appropriation of models of complexity from mathematics and the natural sciences, without regard to the differences as well as continuities between the natural and social worlds. In particular, this may ignore the meaningfulness of the social world and the scope for agents to engage to respond to complexity in different ways.

It follows that we should distinguish complexity in general from specific modes of complexity. The former serves to identify common features of all complex systems and their implications for the dynamics of such systems. These common features include non-linearity, scale dependence, recursiveness, sensitivity to initial conditions, and feedback. Even at this level of analysis, complexity can be studied in many ways, including through algorithmic, deterministic and aggregative analyses [8]. Moreover, social scientists must move from 'complexity in general' as a rational abstraction to study specific modes of complexity in the social world and their interaction with the natural world. We should also recognise that some systems are more complex than others, and that systems may become more or less complex. Such considerations pose interesting problems for the governance of complexity.

What is governance?

Governance is another polyvalent concept. It can refer to all possible modes of co-ordination of complex and reciprocally interdependent activities or operations, as well as to a specific form of such coordination. The most commonly identified modes of coordination are the anarchy of the market, imperative coordination, reflexive self-organisation, and solidarity. In each case, successful coordination depends on the performance of complementary activities and operations by other actors, whose pursuit of their activities and operations depends in turn on such activities and operations being performed elsewhere within the relevant social ensemble. Governance in the narrow sense used here refers to reflexive self-organisation.

Experience shows that all forms of governance are prone to failure. This is reflected in attempts to redesign governance mechanisms and in the recurrent switching among different modes of governance. It is also reflected theoretically in studies of market failure, state failure, failures of collective action based on solidarity and, more recently, failures of reflexive self-organisation. In all cases, despite significant differences between their respective modes of complexity reduction, the continuing excess or surplus of complexity in the real world is a major cause for failure. This explains the growing interest in forms of governance that can integrate the phenomenon of complexity more explicitly, reflexively and, it is hoped, effectively. This holds especially for the trust placed in reflexive self-organisation.

Four factors have been suggested that affect the capacity to build effective self-reflexive governance mechanisms [6]:

1. Simplifying models and practices that reduce the complexity of the world, but have sufficient variety to be congruent with real world processes and to remain relevant to governance objectives. These models should simplify the world without neglecting significant side effects, interdependencies and emerging problems.
2. Developing the capacity for dynamic interactive learning about various causal processes and forms of interdependence, attributions of responsibility and

capacity for actions, and possibilities of coordination in a complex, turbulent environment. This is enhanced when actors can switch among modes of governance to facilitate more effective responses to internal and/or external turbulence.

3. Building methods for coordinating actions among social forces with different identities, interests and meaning systems, over different spatio-temporal horizons and over different domains of action. This depends on self-reflexive self-organisation to sustain exchange, hierarchy, negotiation or solidarity, as well as on the nature of the coordination problems engendered by operating over different scales and time horizons.

4. Establishing a common worldview for individual action and stabilising key players' orientations, expectations and rules of conduct. This permits a more systematic review and assessment of problems and potentials, resource availability and requirements, and the demands of negative and positive coordination.

Nonetheless, self-reflexive organisation also fails. Among the reasons for this are the inadequacy of the definition of the object(s) of governance, the general turbulence of environment, the time required for continuing dialogue, the existence of competing governance projects for same object of governance, and the specific dilemmas in particular forms of governance arrangement. Given that all forms of governance fail, one response has been meta-governance, i.e. the attempt to re-balance modes of governance to ensure more effective switching and joint governance solutions.

Meta-governance failure and beyond

However, given that all forms of governance fail, it is hardly surprising that meta-governance is also failure prone. This could lead to a fatalistic, passive resignation; a stoical, ritualistic approach; self-deluding denial and/or the spinning of failure as success; or cynical opportunism as some actors exit when ahead, leaving others to carry the costs. To avoid such outcomes, three inter-related strategies can be recommended:

1. Deliberate cultivation of a flexible repertoire (requisite variety) of responses.
2. Self-conscious monitoring and reflexivity about governance, its objects, and its outcomes.
3. Self-reflexive 'irony', whereby participants in governance recognise the risks of failure but proceed as if success were possible.

First, the need for flexible 'requisite variety' (with its informational, structural and functional redundancies) is based on recognition that complexity excludes simple governance solutions. Instead, effective governance requires a combination of mechanisms and strategies oriented to the complexities of the object to be governed. Combining strategies and tactics reduces the likelihood of failure, enabling their re-balancing in the face of governance failure and turbulence in the governance environment. Maintaining requisite variety may seem inefficient in economising terms because it introduces slack or waste. But it also provides major sources of flexibility in the face of failure [9]. For, if every mode of economic and political co-ordination is failure-prone, if not failure-laden, longer-term success in coordination depends on the capacity to switch modes as the limits of any one mode become evident.

Second, complexity requires that reflexive observers recognise that they cannot fully understand what they are observing and must make contingency plans for the unexpected. This involves inquiring in the first instance into the material, social and discursive construction of possible objects of governance, and reflecting on why this rather than another object of governance is dominant, hegemonic or naturalised. It requires thinking critically about the strategically selective implications of adopting one or another definition of a specific object of governance and its properties, and, *a fortiori*, of the choice of modes of governance, participants in the governance process, and so forth. Thus, reflexivity involves the ability and commitment to uncover and make explicit one's intentions, projects and actions, their conditions of possibility, and what would be an acceptable outcome in the case of incomplete success. It involves cultivating the ability to learn about them, critique them, and act on any lessons. Applied to meta-governance, this means comparing the effects of failure/inadequacies in markets, government, self-organisation and solidarity, and regularly re-assessing how far current actions are producing desired outcomes. This requires monitoring mechanisms, modulating mechanisms, and a willingness to re-evaluate objectives. And it requires learning about how to learn reflexively. There is a general danger of infinite regress here, of course, but this can be limited provided that reflexivity is combined with the other two principles.

Third, given 'the centrality of failure and the inevitability of incompleteness' [10], how should actors approach the likelihood of failure? The intellectual and practical stance recommended here is that of 'romantic public irony'. To defend this, I distinguish irony from four other responses to governance failure: fatalism, stoicism, denial and cynicism (see above). In contrast to fatalists, stoics, those in denial and cynics, ironists are sceptical and romantic. Recognising the inevitable incompleteness of attempts at governance (whether through the market, imperative coordination or reflexive self-organisation), they adopt a satisficing approach. Ironists accept incompleteness and failure as essential features of social life, but continue to act as if completeness and success were possible. The ironist must simplify a complex, contradictory and changing reality in order to be able to act, knowing full well that any such simplification distorts reality and, worse, that such simplifying distortions can sometimes generate failure as well as enhance the chances of success. In short, even as they expect failure, they act as if they intend to succeed. Moreover, following the law of requisite variety, they must be prepared to change the modes of governance as appropriate.

Complicating matters further, a 'double irony' is present in public romantic irony. For the public romantic ironist recognises the likelihood of failure, but chooses to act on the assumption that success is still possible – thereby 'thinking one thing and doing another'. And, faced with the likelihood of failure, a romantic public ironist chooses her mode of failure. One cannot choose to succeed completely and permanently in a complex world; but one can choose how to fail. This makes it imperative to choose wisely! Given the main alternatives (markets, imperative co-ordination, self-organisation and solidarity) and what we know about how and why they fail, the best chance of reducing the likelihood of failure is to draw on the collective intelligence of stakeholders and other relevant partners in a form of participatory democracy. This does not exclude resorting to other forms of co-ordination, but it does require that the scope granted to the market mechanism, the exercise of formal authority or solidarity is subject as far as possible to decision through forms of participatory governance that aim to balance efficiency, effectiveness and democratic accountability. Key substantive outcomes to be added here include sustainable development, the prioritisation of social justice, and respect for difference. In this sense, public romantic irony is the best mechanism for working out which modes of governance to resort to in particular situations and when collibration is required. It is not the only method to be adopted in all and every situation.

In conclusion, effective governance in the face of complexity requires a commitment to meta-governance rather than relying on just one mode of governance. Romantic public irony, combined with participatory governance, is the best means to optimise the governance of complexity because it recognises the complexity of governance. It also subordinates the roles of market forces, top-down command (especially through the state) and solidarity (with its risk of localism and/or tribalism) to the overall logic of participatory governance. Thus, although some theorists of governance rightly emphasise that governance takes place in the shadow of hierarchy, this should be understood in terms of a democratically accountable, socially inclusive hierarchy organised around the problematic of responsible meta-governance rather than unilateral and top-down command. This places issues of constitutional design at the heart of debates on the future of governance and meta-governance.

Complexity and the bloggers: the rise of the blogosphere

Kingsley Dennis

In this section I describe how newly emerging technologies of information and communication sharing are contributing to a shift in social dynamics of presence and action. The focus will be on blogging specifically, and I will draw from the dynamics of the complexity sciences to show how social information-sharing, non-localised formations/movements are beginning to infringe, influence and change the behaviours of social practice.

The increasing ubiquitous nature of information access is a core component to complex systems and an essential ingredient to the rapid expansion of socio-cultural interactions. The emerging social complexity, I argue, is more unpredictable, rapid, dynamic, and with greater capacity for morphing and transmuting into networks of action.

By looking at the practices of mobile communication through blogging (personal websites), I examine how social collectives of information-sharing individuals both form, and disband, collective groupings in a way that transcends the more traditional local affinities, in order to respond to immediate external events. By doing this I show that an understanding of the complexity sciences can help to illuminate some of the emerging trends of non-localised civil movements that are forming in relation to our mobile information technologies.

Rise of the blogosphere

The term 'weblog', coined by Jorn Barger in December 1997, has been defined as:

> 'Weblogs, also known as blogs, are regularly updated websites or parts of websites, with entries, or posts, in chronological order. Blogs require very little technical skill to maintain, and companies such as Blogger and LiveJournal offer simple tools for hosting weblogs. A person who keeps a weblog is called a blogger. Weblog posts usually link to news articles, other weblogs, or other websites, and are accompanied by the blogger's commentary, which can include personal opinions, factual corrections, and anything in between' [11].

Anyone can start a weblog, it does not require any tech-knowledge or sophistication as it comes as a ready-made template. Once a person registers[3], they are able to start publishing straight away: web-publishing at one's fingertips.

What makes the weblog more dynamic and durable than the homepage is its fluidity: it is updated almost daily (sometimes several times daily); it is easily modified as it uses a downloadable template; and it adapts to the newly arriving information like a conversation. What makes it so easy for the amateur to link, trackback and forge connections in such a heavily dense blogosphere? One of the answers comes in the form of collective tools: *syndication*. A technology known as RSS is beginning to transform how people can customise how Internet content is to be delivered. Initially RSS stood for RDF site summary, or rich site summary. Now it is more generally known as really simple syndication. Again, with reference to the Aula gathering:

> 'It is a format used to syndicate web content of news sites, community sites, and personal weblogs. It can be thought of as a way of subscribing to websites. RSS makes it easier to keep up with favourite sites, and at the same time it is a convenient way of ensuring that others can keep up with one's own site. The RSS feed contains headlines, a link to the actual item, and optionally a description or summary of the update' [11].

What RSS allows is for the user to customise the delivery of their Internet content. It is a syndication ability that allows readers of blogs, websites, news sites, and other pages in which they have an interest, to enable their computers to retrieve the latest updates to these pages and deliver them to the reader in the form of an indexed content-cataloguing. Thus, on one page a reader can see the latest headlines, or tag words, to a hundred or more of the Internet pages to which that reader regularly follows. From there the reader can see a brief summary of the updated page, and has a link that takes them directly to it if they so wish. Control of information flow is being shifted over to the user/reader: this is a dramatic shift away from the norms of traditional media. With the proliferation of rapid linking between blogsites, coupled with the conversational search engines such as Technorati, as well as the customised RSS content feeds, information is spreading, being networked, stored and used, at increased speed and complexity. The concept of self-reflexivity, and feedback monitoring, is almost second nature to regular bloggers, and also to others who deal in peer-to-peer information sharing.

---

3 This is usually for free, although some companies are now charging a minimal fee for upkeep and support.

The rise to prominence of the bloggers came principally after 9/11 and the subsequent 'War on Terror'. By 2002, many of the well-known bloggers were supporting the US-led strategies to confront Iraq and the controversy about weapons of mass destruction, largely because they came from prominent politically right orientated sites such as 'Instapundit'. The term then used – 'war bloggers' – was broadened to include all those bloggers whose main focus at the time was the war in Iraq, irrespective of their political position. By the spring of 2003, *Forbes Magazine* used 'war blogger' in this larger sense when listing the 'best warblogs' (http://en.wikipedia.org/wiki/Blogging). Since then, blogging, or the blogosphere, has become a mix of debates and issues. Bloggers are now distributed among all political, racial, religious and ethnic positions.

Weblogs are nowadays noted for being among the first to cite, break, disseminate and cover or criticise the latest news. Some of the more famous blogs that cover the Iraqi situation are: 'The Baghdad Blogger' (http://raedinthemiddle.blogspot.com/); 'Baghdad Burning' (http://riverbendblog.blogspot.com/); and 'Back to Iraq' (http://www.back-to-iraq.com/). There are literally thousands of blogs covering such issues as the invasion of Iraq, so it would be beyond scope to go into such detailed lists. As of January 2006, Technorati cites over 75,000 new weblogs being created each day – one roughly every second. Technorati is currently watching 30.3 million blogs and tracking 2.1 billion links (11 March 2006). By the time I write these words, the previous figures are already out of date. The blogosphere moves fast, and so does its news.

Blogosphere networks

It is estimated that about 11% (approximately 50 million) of Internet users are regular blog readers. Active bloggers, meanwhile, update their blogs regularly, to the tune of more than 275,000 posts daily, or about 11,000 updates an hour [12]. It is also a known feature that blog-traffic increases sharply when certain web news-events occur: as in the London bombings of July 2005.

Not only do blog-sites peak at particular newsworthy events, they also cluster around the more well-known or prestigious sites; what can be called the blog-attractors. This is a feature of the nature of networks. Network researcher Albert-Laszlo Barabasi considers networks to be the precursor to any complex system [13]. In the research that Barabasi undertook, he found that networks start with an array of nodes that facilitate links between them. However, after a 'critical number of links', particular nodes will become stronger attractors, i.e. attracting more links to them than other nodes. This will in turn transform those specific nodes into hubs, or clusters. These clusters then attract further links which then strengthen their own attraction. Barabasi states that such 'connectors-nodes with an anonymously large number of links are present in very diverse complex systems, ranging from the economy to the cell' [13].

Bernardo Huberman, researching networks at Hewlett-Packard, has formulated a *power law* that can adequately describe the distribution between 'the number of pages per site, and also the number of links emanating from a site or coming to it' [14]. From what appears to be a pattern of genuine non-random user-response, a website becomes initially more popular and then begins to add on more links, and 'the more links a site has, the more visible it becomes and the more new links it will get' [14]. This is such that a site will self-organise its growth through its connectivity with other linked sites. The bottom-up geography displayed by the new mobile web communications show a shift towards clusters of blog-sites. According to Technorati, the blogging search site, the top-ranking site – Boing Boing – has 19,265 links (at 16 January 2006), thus making it the strongest blog-attractor and thus a leading node in the blogosphere network. These major blog-attractors then demonstrate that the blogosphere, like other complex systems such as the economy and the cell, work within a network topology that is the basis upon which complex systems operate [15]. Further, the blogosphere maintains its own far-from-equilibrium and dynamic random order through the constant open flow of information.

In the blogosphere then, as in networks, the pattern follows that of the scale-free network. Here, particular nodes will become stronger attractors, i.e. attracting more links to them than other nodes. This will in turn transform those specific nodes into hubs, or clusters. These clusters then attract further links, which then strengthen their own attraction. The blogosphere, the Internet, networks and complex systems show patterns that form what has been termed as 'scale-free'.

Such network-presence is becoming increasingly influential in the political domain. An internet study on the French European Union referendum of 29 May 2005 by two researchers at the University of Technology of Compiègne (http://www.utc.fr/rtgi/index.php?rubrique=1&sousrubrique=0&study=constitution) discovered some interesting correlations. Of the original 12,000 sites that were scanned, finally only 295 web/blog sites that specifically dealt with the referendum were chosen. Of those sites, 79 were supporting the 'Yes' campaign, whereas 161 were on the side of 'No'; this constituting an imbalance of 67% of sites for 'Non', with only 33% for the 'Oui' camp. The analysis further showed that the density of links within the network of 'No' sites were of higher density than those within the 'Yes' cluster. Of the 161 'No' sites, there were 432 internal linkages between them, with there being only 33 links externally to some of the 'Yes' sites. In contrast, of the 79 'Yes' sites there were only 159 links between them, yet with 41, an interesting comparably higher percentage of links, going into the 'No' sites. This again showed that the information-networks formed within the web/blogosphere of the victorious side is the one that has a higher density of internal linkages between its parts, and lesser influence coming in from external sites. Again, such information is inclusive when forming conclusions about the role of such phenomena on the eventual outcome of such events. Saying this, it does posit a suggestion that the complex structure of how information is disseminated may relate to physical behaviour such as voting patterns. Such complex collectives can be seen to be efficient in getting their point across.

What can complexity tell us?

Sporadic social movements are emerging in diverse geographical regions: they represent self-organising complex systems based upon networks of mediated mobile information. These groupings/clusters are self-organising, dynamic, far-from-equilibrium and maintain themselves through information flows, thus exhibiting characteristics that can ally them with the complex systems of the complexity sciences [16]. What is beginning to emerge are complex collectives of information-utilising human agents within co-presence and action. This relationship with information flows increasingly puts an emphasis upon mobility and movement, spontaneity, and more dynamic forms of social relations: signs that point towards new reconfigurations within the scapes and flows of a global complexity [7].

The information flows emerging in this environment are the many-to-many (increasingly referred to as 'peer-to-peer') that invests the user(s) with an increased sense of autonomy in terms of what information is received, used and transmitted. This new format provides opportunities and electronic proximities for grassroots activism in such areas as 'gathering and disseminating alternative and more democratic news; creating virtual public spheres where citizens debate the issues that concern democratic societies; and organizing collective political action' [17]. What appears to be materialising at this stage of our global communications are pockets, or rather subsets, of systemic behaviour, coordinated by mobile information communications. And they do not necessarily need to be coordinated throughout, if the initial stimulus is sufficient to sustain a continued flow of information and messaging. It is for such reasons as these that I am arguing that complex systemic behaviour as manifested within the complexity sciences can, and does, have a place when modelling these features of emerging mobilised crowds and informationally activated individuals.

The World Wide Web is still an immature phenomenon, approximately a decade in existence, and still in its infancy of potential development and capacity. Those Net-literate individuals who are aware and clued into using a combination of emerging technologies are the early-users that are forming and participating in these sub-groups of complex, information-rich systems that manifest the individuals (parts) as active agents. What the future of this phenomenon will be is still undecided. In the next few years these 'self-organized, citizen-centric movements enabled by smart mob media will either demonstrate real political influence...or recede as a utopian myth of days gone by' [17].

This section is a beginning in examining the rise of the blogosphere as an example of such 'citizen-centric movements' that have made an influence upon political events.

Complexity, cities and social action: a consideration of the implications of the complexity frame of reference for praxis
David Byrne

> Praxis – the willed action by which a theory or philosophy is translated into social reality – related to the classical Greek notion of pragmata which implies that human actors must do something.

I have a longstanding engagement with 'action-research' both as a practitioner and as an academic reflecting on the implications of action-research for the nature of social science as a social practice. This dual engagement has been conducted at the interface among the fields of social policy and urban studies and the discipline of sociology, with particular reference to sociology's methodological programme. 'Complexity theory' has provided a way of understanding both the nature of the systems with which I have been engaged as an action-researcher and, taken together with a critical realist approach to causation, an answer to the crucial methodological issue of action-research: how can we generalise from this complex and developing experience to any other context? In other words, how can we provide some sort of guidance as to 'what works'? Let me be clear here. When we assert that we have some way of saying 'what works', then we are in the business of prediction. We are committing to the central project of modernity – the organisation of knowledge as the basis of an effective technology of change.

Cilliers has identified the issues that a responsible postmodernist turn might assert would derive from this position in a commentary on Derrida:

> *'The immense gain of the notion of difference is that it reminds us that not only the past has to be considered when we try to establish the meaning of (say) an event, but that since we cannot fully predict the effects of this event, the future has to be considered as well, despite the fact that we might have no idea what the future might be. Now, instead of throwing up his hands, and declaring that in such a case it is impossible to talk about meaning, and that therefore anything goes, Derrida insists that we should take responsibility for this unknowable future'* [18].

The great advantage of a complexity take is that it denies that the future is unknowable even if it is not simply determined. The analytical programme of determining simple and exact causation provides a mode of prediction where it is applicable, which works in a straightforward fashion. Knowledge of initial conditions and of universal covering law enables us to say if we do this, then this will happen. Derrida's take is that we have no idea of what the future will be. Complexity – understood as an ontological specification of the nature of complex systems coupled with a realist conception of contingent and complex causation – allows us to say what the future might be and what future comes to be depends on what we do. In complex systems, future trajectories are multiple but not infinite. Things may stay much the same. Things may change. There are a range of possible future changed states. Which state comes to be depends – is determined by – the interaction of a set of control parameters in which human agency, both collective and individual, both purposeful and not purposeful, plays a crucial part.

And complexity as a scientific approach offers us something else. It offers us a way in which we might understand how our actions can be shaped in given contexts to produce particular outcomes. However, this knowledge will never work if it is considered as something that can be externally constructed outwith the systems with which it is engaged. Indeed, a central argument here will be that knowledge that purports to be external, general and objective will always be engaged with social systems, but will be so engaged in the interests of dominant elites. There is an alternative way of doing things, a way that outside the domain of its political application in Brazil has all too often been 'employed' as a radical rhetorical colouring for an at best banal but more often deceptive set of practices of incorporating community work 'in and for the state'. However, it is in origin a radical practical resolution of the dilemmas of reason in modernity, a resolution moreover which is certainly eclectic but is also sophisticated in its engagement with those dilemmas, and which draws on a range of radical critiques and practices in developing an original model for real social engagement. This is Paulo Freire's programme of conscientisation.

Let me use Crotty's excellent gloss to indicate the nature of this project:

'To denote the fact that the dynamic structure of consciousness is inseparable from the objects that inform it, in other words that "authentic thought-language" is generated in and out of a dialectical relationship between human beings and their concrete historical and cultural reality (Freire 1972b: p.13), Freire uses the word employed by Brentano, Husserl and the phenomenonologists generally – intentionality. The intentionality of consciousness means that consciousness is never a mere reflection of material reality but is a reflection upon [original emphasis] material reality (1972b: p.53). Consciousness is already an active intervention into reality. Critical reflection is already action. …. Authentic action and reflection are indissolubly united, therefore. This is Freire's understanding of praxis [original emphasis]. It is "reflection and action upon the world in order to transform it" (Freire 1972a: p.28). True praxis can never be merely cerebral. It must involve action. Nor can it be limited to mere activism. It must include serious reflection (1972a: pp.40–41). Freire regards reflection without action as sheer verbalism, "armchair revolution", whereas action without reflection is "pure activism", that is action for action's sake' [19].

Of course, the phenomenological/existential programme has always been – to use Gramsci's useful term – a programme of and for traditional intellectuals. In contrast Freire argues, very much in the spirit of Gramsci's assertion, that 'all men [*sic*] are intellectuals' for a set of practices which are essentially organic and transformational. The key process in this is conscientisation, which:

'is more than taking consciousness, because being aware is a normal way of being human. It involves to analyse. It is a way of seeing the world in a precise or almost precise way. It is a way of seeing how society works. It is a better way of understanding the set of problems, a question of power. How to obtain power, what means not having power. Finally, it involves a deeper reading of the reality and of the common sense, and beyond it' [20].

Freire developed his ideas in contexts of real material exploitation and deprivation – even today in the Brazilian northeast millions of people live with a diet that is absolutely inadequate – whereas we operate in a context in which poverty has to be understood as relative and most people have resources that enable high levels of personal and familial consumption; but the fundamental inequalities of power remain the same, even if perhaps the key issues for us are retention of the egalitarian gains of a social democratic past and attention to an ecological future, rather than contemporary gross exploitation and material deprivation in our own lives. Of course, the lives of others do matter and the politics of recognition of that point are perhaps the liveliest domain of real engagement in the contemporary UK.

The key process here is dialogue in participatory research. Sue Sohng defines this process thus:

'Participatory research challenges practices that separate the researcher from the researched and promotes the forging of a partnership between researchers

and the people under study ... Both researcher and participant are actors in the investigative process, influencing the flow, interpreting the content, and sharing options for action. ... The result of this kind of activity is living knowledge that may get translated into action ... ' [21].

What complexity brings to participatory research is a frame of reference that indicates that a different world is possible, – with 'world' understood at whatever level is relevant for participants in the process and as they develop that understanding – and demonstrates that critical collective and dialogical reflection will enable us to grasp how history might be shaped in particular ways in a given socio-historical context. Essentially, what complexity offers is a way of understanding histories – the plural is very important – as a method of shaping futures. The owl of Minerva can be given a boot up the backside to move in a particular direction.

There is an interesting issue as to how complexity methods can enter into and inform dialogical participatory research. At the most basic level the idea of social systems as complex is cognate with 'lay' understandings of the nature of social causation and social change. This means that people can draw on their repertoire of current understanding to address these issues. It is also worth noting that many methods of representing complex systems and change in those systems are inherently graphical. People seem to have an innate ability to grasp visual representations, especially dynamic visual representations. Moreover, complexity can be represented through narrative. Of course, the whole point of dialogue is that the knowledge non-technical participants have also enters into the formation of account. The ways in which this can be done through narrative are relatively clear. It can also be done through visual images [22]. In general, there is a multiplicity of perspectives available for representation of complex systems and their trajectories.

However, the key thing to determine is 'what makes a difference?'. This is where systematic comparative analysis comes into its own. I have written at length about this elsewhere but here will merely content myself with asserting that figurational techniques, based on careful qualitative work in reflexive dialogue – by which is meant both the elicitation of information and the taking back of accounts for further discussion – has much to offer in action-research contexts.

Action-research has developed as a research practice in a range of applied fields in the social sciences, but the implications of the process have not informed meta-methodological debate. Original interventions in action-research argued for strict experimental designs, but under the influence of practice and of the pedagogical theories of Paulo Freire there has been a general shift towards dialogical modes of engagement with social actors in the research field. This means that scientists – in the Gulbenkian Commission's sense of this role as generators of ' ... systematic secular knowledge about reality that is somehow validated empirically' [4] – do not confine their engagement with social actors to the elicitation of information, but in the process of research feedback in which there is a dialogue both as to the validity of account and as to its implications for practice. This has much in common, although there does not seem to be much if any cross-referencing, with integrative methods as proposed by Lemon *et al.* [23] which is explicitly complexity based. The point about action-research is that it takes the process of reflexivity out of the epistemological ghetto and into social life. It is reflexivity that leads not to relativistic passivity but rather to engagement in action. In this respect it meets Paul Cilliers' requirement that those who wish to engage with complex social systems must, ethically, do so from within those systems. There are many contexts in which action-research is applicable. One of the most obvious is in relation to the planning processes which determine the future trajectories of city regions. A technicist/scientistic version of complexity will work for elites in such processes. A dialogical version of complexity has the potential for working very differently.

Let me conclude by expanding on the tension between technicist complexity for elites and dialogical complexity for the 'popular masses' in relation to the future trajectories of city regions. The key theme here is the difference between consultation/implementation participation on the one hand and genuine participatory democracy on the other. Those who manage governance in post-industrial cities – essentially urban regimes in which there is a mix of public and private sector representation – have a real need for information about real learning feedback, both about the whole social environment and especially about the social processes of urban systems in areas with which they no longer have any direct experience based on real contacts. Under effective democratic processes, especially in the high period of Fordist capitalism from World War II until about 1980, locally elected municipal representatives were a key source of such information. In post-democratic market capitalism that conduit is largely ineffective. So mechanisms of consultation and participation in implementation have been developed. However, these are very different from real participatory democracy in which alternative futures based on very different real interests become the basis of political contestation. Effectively, consultation is never about what should be done but only about how to do it once the key strategic decisions have been taken. Action-research directed towards establishing the range of alternative futures inevitably contributes to conflict because it establishes more than one possibility as the basis towards which public policy should be directed. The neo-liberal consensus that is the essence of contemporary politics will be replaced by real ideological – ideologies are ideas about power and interests – dispute. The management of urban systems is all about planning. A dialogical conception of action-research in relation to complexity makes the questions: planning for what? planning for whom? central to policy. It will bring politics back in, and in my concluding view about time too!

References

1. Urry J. The Complexity turn. *Theory, Culture & Society* **22** (5): 1–14. 2005.
2. Thrift N. The place of complexity. *Theory, Culture & Society* **16** (3): 31–69. 1999.
3. Thrift N. The place of complexity. *Theory, Culture & Society* **16** (3): 31–69. 1999.
4. Gulbenkian-Commission. *Open the Social Sciences: Report on the restructuring of the social sciences*. Stanford: Stanford University Press. 1996.
5. Waldrop M. *Complexity: The emerging science at the edge of order and chaos*. London: Viking. 1992.
6. Jessop B. The governance of complexity and the complexity of governance. In: *Beyond Markets and Hierarchy* (eds A. Amin and J. Hausner), pp.111–147. Chelmsford: Edward Elgar. 1997.
7. Urry J. *Global Complexity*. Cambridge: Polity Press. 2003.
8. Rescher N. *Complexity: A philosophical overview*. New Brunswick: Transaction Books. 1998.

9. Grabher G. *Lob der Verschwendung*. Berlin: Sigma. 1994.

10. Malpas J., Wickham G. Governance and Failure: on the limits of sociology. *Australia and New Zealand Journal of Society* **31** (3): 37–50. 1995.

11. Ahtisaari M., Engestrom J., Nieminen A. (editors). *Exposure – From friction to freedom*. I-Print.

12. McGann R. The blogosphere by the numbers. http://www.clickz.com/stats/sectors/traffic_patterns/article.php/3438891; 22 November 2004.

13. Barabasi A.-L. *Linked*. London: Plume. 2003.

14. Huberman B. *The Laws of the Web: Patterns in the ecology of information*. Cambridge, MA: MIT Press. 2001.

15. Prigogine I. *The End of Certainty*. New York: The Free Press. 1997.

16. Prigogine I, Nicolis G. *Self-Organization in Non-Equilibrium Systems*. New York: John Wiley. 1977.

17. Rheingold H. From the screen to the streets. http://www.inthesetimes.com/comments.php?id=414_0_1_0_C accessed 22 March 2005.

18. Cilliers P. *Complexity and Postmodernism*. London: Routledge. 1998.

19. Crotty M. *The Foundations of Social Research*. London: Sage. 1998.

20. Torres A.C. A pedagogia política de Paulo Freire. In: *Paulo Freire: Política e pedagogia* (eds M.W. Apple and A. Nóvoa), pp.235–244. Porto: Porto Editora. Universidade de Lisboa: Portugal. 1998.

21. Sohng S.L. Participatory research and community organizing. A working paper presented at The New Social Movement and Community Organizing Conference. University of Washington, Seattle, WA, 1–3 November 1995. http://www.interweb-tech.com/nsmnet/docs/sohng.htm.

22. Byrne D.S., Doyle A. The visual and the verbal – the interaction of images and discussion in exploring cultural change. In: *Using Visual Methods* (eds C. Knowles and P. Sweetman). London: Routledge. 2005.

23. Lemon M. (editor). *Exploring Environmental Change Using an Integrative Method*. Amsterdam: Gordon and Breach. 1999.

Further reading

Byrne D.S. Complexity, configurations and cases. *Theory, Culture & Society* **22** (5): 95–111. 2005.

Estrela M.T. Reflective practice and conscientisation. *Pedagogy, Culture & Society* **7** (2): 1999.

Flyvbjerg B. *Making Social Science Matter*. Cambridge: Cambridge University Press. 2001.

Gerhardt H.P. Paulo Freire. *Prospects 2000* **XXIII** (3/4): 439–458. 1993.

Holland J.H. *Emergence*. Reading, MA: Addison-Wesley. 1998.

Ragin C.C. *The Comparative Method*. Berkeley: University of California Press. 1987.

Ragin C.C. *Fuzzy-Set Social Science*. Chicago: Chicago University Press. 2000.

Reed M., Harvey D.H. The new science and the old: complexity and realism in the social sciences. *Journal for the Theory of Social Behaiour* **22**: 356–379. 1992.

Shargel E.I., Dwyer M. On the road from Husserl to Freire. *Philosophy of Education* **2000**: 189–191. 2000.

CHAPTER 11

Conclusion: making complexity real

Jan Bogg and Robert Geyer

As you 'set sail' on your own complexity journey, an important quality in any change agent, researcher or leader, as we advocated in our *Times Higher Education Supplement* article [1], involves engaging in considering paradigm shifts and new ways of working and looking at the world. There is a poem by Janet Kalven, particularly relevant to thinking outside the box:

> *You have set a sail on another ocean*
> *Without star or compass*
> *Going where the argument leads*
> *Shattering the certainties of centuries*

> JANET KALVEN
> *Respectable Outlaw*

In open evolutionary systems where the components are strongly interrelated, self-organising and dynamic, each system must evolve in relation to the larger environment in which it operates:

> *'The most important characteristic of the Eastern world view, one could almost say the essence of it – is the awareness of the unity and mutual interrelation of all things and events, the experience of all phenomena in the world as manifestations of a basic oneness. All things are seen as interdependent and inseparable parts of this cosmic whole; as different manifestations of the same ultimate reality.'*

> FRITJOF CAPRA, *The Tao of Physics*

To survive, the system must change and adapt. This is not a new phenomenon: as the Buddha noted, everything changes, with impermanence being the reality:

> *'The world is continuous flux and is impermanent.'*

Complexity science represents a growing body of interdisciplinary knowledge about the structure, behaviour and dynamics of change in complex adaptive systems. This has numerous applications, including science, society, healthcare and economics. The authors of papers in this book have all demonstrated how complexity can help us to understand and work with change. As we have seen, complexity exists at the edge of chaos, as a dynamic state between order and chaos. In our daily lives, people use the words 'chaos' and 'complexity' to understand and describe events. This relates to common issues such as 'chaos in the classroom', the 'complexity of patient care' or even 'national security is a complex situation'.

This has implications for complexity researchers in terms of the use of words such as 'complex' or 'complexity'. What do the words mean? Do individuals know or even understand what we are talking about when we refer to our 'complexity-based' research? What of the future for complexity-based research and ensuring that our research has practical currency and application to real-world problems? Application in the health sector can be used as an example of application to 'real-world' problems. As has been suggested:

> 'The NHS is the epitome of a complex adaptive system. Such systems do not always respond well to mechanistic formulae'.
>
> DAVID FILLIGHAM, *Director,*
> *National Health Service Modernistation Agency*
> (*Health Services Journal* 7 (2): 27. 2002.)

Moore [2] commented that innovation is so difficult in the National Health Service (NHS) because of attitudes and infrastructure. He went on to state that:

> 'The major problem lies in a combination of attitudes and infrastructure, in other words, what people are willing to adopt and what support there is to adopt it. Another problem is the conventional approach to evidence based medicine that if applied uncritically can lead to flawed assumptions about efficacy of new treatments.'

Moore suggests that attitudes related to enquiry and commitment to improving patient care, in combination with government support and organisational factors such as flexibility and ensuring that the patient is central in decision making, are needed to foster innovation. Using a complexity model would facilitate this.

Analysing clinical care using complexity theory draws many parallels with the holistic model of healthcare. Holistic healthcare is an integrated approach to healthcare that treats the 'whole' person, not simply symptoms and disease, with mind and body viewed as integrated and inseparable. Treatment from a holistic healthcare perspective involves more than identifying an illness and routine treatment: the healthcare professional considers the illness, the patient's lifestyle, socio-economic factors, the external environment, health beliefs and attitudes when treating the patient. This concept of holistic healthcare has increased in popularity with the public in recent years, as mind and body are viewed as related in health and illness. Healthcare practitioners are also increasingly starting to consider such influences in the research area of psychoneuroimmunology. That is the complex relationship and influencing factors of psychology, neurology and immunological factors or 'mind and body connections' in mortality and morbidity.

Complexity science can be used to understand and develop models of co-ordinated care pathways. This principle of analysing and understanding the functioning relationships between the interacting agents in a clinical scenario, in order to try and improve coordination of care, can be considered applicable to all clinical situations involving complex patients, including those with diabetes or HIV. To improve care coordination involves understanding the functioning of the relationships between the interacting agents. Therefore, the communication between the different healthcare providers needs to be assessed to determine communication and the barriers and drivers to effective communication, before developing protocols to improve care coordination.

Recent research by Matlow *et al.* [3] discusses how the principles of complexity science can be applied to improve the coordination of care for complex paediatric patients. The main issue raised by the paper was how lack of communication between families, specialists and other service providers resulted in uncoordinated care, causing frustration for the patient and family and inefficient and poor-quality patient care. Coordinated healthcare for paediatric patients included itemising and planning treatment strategies, coordinating visits with sub-specialists, organising care to avoid duplication of diagnostic tests and services, sharing information between healthcare professionals and patients, reassessing and readjusting the care plan on a regular basis.

Using complexity science to improve care coordination involved understanding the functioning of the relationships between the interacting agents. Therefore, it was recognised that communication between the different healthcare providers should be assessed to evaluate communication and identify barriers to good communication.

The most valuable asset of the NHS is its workforce, and complexity has a crucial role to play in understanding the relationships involved in workforce issues. Complexity has provided a useful framework for research in this area, especially in planning for change. For example, Jan Bogg's Breaking Barriers in the Workplace project (http://www.liv.ac.uk/climpsy/breakingbarriers) at the University of Liverpool is using complexity as a framework for understanding the barriers and drivers to career progression in the bio- and health sciences sector. The project methodology uses qualitative and quantitative methods, and the participants in different phases range from recently qualified to Department of Health leaders. So far, phase 1 [4] analysed data on 1,600 participants, and the current phase 2 [5] have conducted over 140 one-to-one interviews. Complexity science is crucial in maintaining a balance between order and chaos, in the multiplicity of viewpoints and organisational considerations, and in making sense of the relationships and meanings in terms of policy, procedure and outcomes.

Health has been used as one example of how complexity can be used, its 'real-world currency'. Complexity has many applications, and this book has highlighted some of the excellent work that is making complexity 'real' for people. Real-life applications will ensure that the word 'complexity' has true value and real meaning. Then, as we suggested in the introduction by using the Hawking quotation, the century really will be one of complexity.

> *'I think the next century will be the century of complexity.'*
> STEPHEN HAWKING (2000) *in San Jose Mercury News*

References

1. Bogg J., Geyer R. Outside all the boxes: complexity theory makes room for both Newton and disorder. *Times Higher Education Supplement*, 23 September 2005.
2. Moore B. Why is innovation so difficult in the NHS? *Clinical Discovery*, July 2006. http://www.clinicaldiscovery.com/.
3. Matlow A.G., Wright J.G., Zimmerman B., Thomson K., Valente M. How can the principles of complexity science be applied to improve the coordination of care for complex paediatric patients? *Quality and Safety in Health Care* **15**: 85–88. 2006.
4. Bogg J. Breaking barriers in the workplace project (further details and downloadable executive summary phase 1) http://www.liv.ac.uk/climpsy/breakingbarriers.
5. Bogg J., Sartain S. Barriers and drivers to women's career progression. *Clinical Discovery*. August 2006.

Index